HEAL THY
SOUL!!

.....Naturally with TIPS TO STRENGTHEN YOUR BODY'S WEAKEST LINKS

Roberta T. McClinon

DISCLAIMER

No part of this book may be used or reproduced in any manner whatsoever without the prior written permission except in the case of brief quotations utilized in articles and reviews. The information expressed in this book are not to be taken as medical advice, but rather to represent the author's opinions and are solely for informational and educational purposes. The author is not responsible for any injury or health conditions that may occur through following the programs and information or opinions expressed herein. Dietary information is also only presented for informational purposes only and may not be appropriate for all individuals. Always consult your physician or health care professional before starting any exercise program or changing your diet.

DEDICATION

I dedicate this book, first and foremost to The Most High God whom without I would not be where I am today. Without Him, I could not have overcome the obstacles that were placed in my way but ultimately, become my stepping stones that helped create my passion for helping others change and improve their lives and health for the better.

To my children, James Kendrick, Jr. and Alnisaa Evans, you are my rocks! God blessed me with two of the most wonderful, caring and selfless children on earth. You have been and continue to be my strength. You had to grow up pretty fast when you were young by taking on very adult responsibilities.

You could have become resentful, selfish and uncaring, however, today you continue to look out for my wellbeing and are very nurturing and hands on parents to your children. I believe having to take on such responsibility contributed to the wonderful job you're doing raising my beautiful grandbabies. Although I know you still would have become wonderful people and parents even without having to take care of me while you were young, the challenge of caring for a parent at such a crucial and critical time in your own lives laid the foundation early for you to be nurturers to your own children.

To all my family and friends, who are too numerous to mention and I don't want leave anyone out, thank you for always encouraging and supporting me through everything I have been through. I couldn't have found the courage to keep going in spite of the ups and downs and sometimes the doubts about whether I am doing the right thing in pursuing my passion.

I love and appreciate each and every one of you!

ABOUT THE AUTHOR

Roberta T. McClinon earned her Bachelor of Natural Health and Doctor of Naturopathy degrees from the Clayton College of Natural Health. She is a Registered Certified Reflexologist in the state of Tennessee and received her certification from the International Institute of Reflexology and is also a Reiki II Practitioner. As a motivational speaker and seminar presenter, she loves to share and teach others that they can improve their health and overcome major obstacles just as she has and live a quality life on all levels.

For over 40 years, Roberta has been on a personal and professional journey of wellness. Her own struggles with ill health has been the catalyst for finding her passion to help others to never give up no matter how hard it may seem. But to always take responsibility and do what is in _your_ power to own your health – mentally, physically, spiritually and emotionally. Also, seek the help and support you need to get through and overcome any barriers necessary to achieve your goals.

TABLE OF CONTENTS

INTRODUCTION

When I was looking for a name for my business, I wrote down several potential names I thought would be fitting of what I wanted to represent and came up with the name HEALTHY SOULS. I felt this name summarized everything I wanted to convey to my clients and anyone I came in contact with as well as what I was seeking for myself and my life.

Being HEALTHY was the main objective I had been seeking when working to bring my body back in balance. When you divide the word "healthy", you get "heal" "thy". SOUL – represented the essence of my whole being on all levels – physical, mental, emotional and spiritual.

Exactly what is our SOUL? If we are seeking to heal it, what is wrong with it and why does it need healing, what do you do? I'm sure you're expecting me to give you a reasonable, intelligent or even a scientific answer to those questions, but I don't have a set answers that is any different than what you may have heard already. I could spend hours researching and quoting from spiritual advisors and experts, scientists and other authorities who would give their thoughts, expertise and opinions. So, I will just give you my intuitive feelings and thoughts on it.

The soul is the essence of who we are. That part of you that exists without your awareness. My first thought of what could be considered the SOUL, came to me when I was around 11 years old. I recall looking in the mirror one day and just wondering how is it that I can think, feel and exist within this space. Where were all the feelings, emotions, thoughts that I had – good or bad –coming from. How did I become this "person" physically with this dark skin, this mouth, these eyes, that nose, that hair – not in an inferior or superior judgmental way, just in a curious wonderment (is that a word? Hhmmm)! Like WOW! Isn't GOD AMAZING!! At the same time, I felt that there was a part of me that was not visible, that could not be touched but was responsible for my existence.

Sure, I knew I came from my parents, but how did I become ME? The essence, the purity, fullness, emptiness of me? Why was I here and not somewhere else – beyond my physical environment? A lot to think about at that age, however, I believe what I was really trying to find and describe was my SOUL.

What I was searching for was everything that came together to give me purpose in this life. So when I think of HEALING MY – THY SOUL, it's all of our experiences in the physical, mental, spiritual and emotional realm. To HEAL it has to come full circle and in balance or at least some sense of fullness and completion to the best degree as possible.

This book is meant to pique your interest and start you to think more about your health and your SOUL in a way that will put YOU in charge of becoming the best you can be with methods and suggestions that you can pick and choose according to your individual needs or desires. It's like going to a restaurant, you can choose your favorite entrée or you can choose individual items "a la carte".

So, how do you begin to determine *your* body's weakest link? Once you know what it is, what do you do about it? How do you strengthen it? What does it involve? How do you heal *your* SOUL?

You may find one link that you want to incorporate and focus solely on that before choosing another. Or you may decide 2 or 3 of them can be easily incorporated into your lifestyle. It's your choice! I will be covering several topics that individually can add health benefits on some level. However, the goal is to incorporate several of these topics and find ways to apply them into your daily lifestyle for long term and long lasting health improvement – part of the completion of your SOUL journey!

The human body is an amazing and wondrous "machine"! Sometimes we forget how amazing and miraculous the human body is! At one time each of us was only a microscopic organism! Too often we take this for granted. *Our* bodies are compared to computers and machines, when in reality *computers and machines* are most likely based on the incredible anatomy and functions of the human body. For example, the CPU (central processing unit) of a computer is the "brain".

> *"I will praise thee; for I am fearfully and wonderfully made; marvelous are thy works; and that my SOUL knoweth right well.*
>
> *My substance was not hid from thee, when I was made in secret, and curiously wrought in the lowest parts of the earth.*
>
> *Thine eyes did see my substance, yet being imperfect; and in thy book all my members were written, which in continuance were fashioned, when as yet there was none of them."*
>
> Psalms 139:14-16

Our bodies are made of different organs, glands, nerves, bones, tissues, muscles, cells and other matter. When viewing the body in its totality it's not possible to understand the inner workings of all that it takes to make and keep this glorious machine functioning – hopefully at its peak performance.

Even with all the knowledge and understanding we have access to, there are potential and probable "malfunctions" that can and do occur inside and outside of our bodies. Some of the "weaknesses" that occur in the body are caused by various functions and circumstances such as heredity, genetics, environment, the natural process of dying off of cells, diet, emotional state, accidents and so on.

Within all its functions the body desires to reach a level of homeostasis or balance. However, sometimes maintaining this balance can be a challenge due to the weaknesses mentioned above. These "weak links" aren't necessarily due to one particular organ or body system but can be caused by several factors.

The links included here are just a short list of choices you can make to keep your body operating at its fullest potential. The human body is a miracle in and of itself. All the functions it is capable of performing have yet to be discovered by man! God in His infinite wisdom has designed us in ways that are absolutely mind blowing.

So at this point we will explore the links that will bring your attention to some factors that may strengthen YOUR body's particular weak link(s) and allow you to take responsibility for those things that you have control over. You should not abandon your doctor or health care professional but help them help you on your SOUL's health journey.

LINK #1

AS A MAN THINKETH, SO IS HE: EMOTIONAL, MENTAL & SPIRITUAL WELL-BEING

To get a true understanding of how to balance the body we must take into account every aspect of who we are. We are not just our physical body. We are also emotional, mental and spiritual beings – a complete SOUL.

With some understanding of the different body systems and body types, what role do emotions play in health? Studies have shown that 80% of physical problems stem from emotional issues. Have you ever heard someone say, "He/she makes me sick!" or "Every time I talk about a certain event or situation, I get a knot in my stomach"? That "physical" response can create illness and dis-ease in the body if not dealt with appropriately.

Many of us may be familiar with the saying "Sticks and Stone May Break My Bones but Words Will Never Hurt Me!". Nothing could be further from the truth. Words CAN HURT YOU! WORDS HAVE MEANING AND POWER! "Sticks & Stones May Break My Bones, But Words Can *DESTROY* Me!" – Emotionally, Mentally, Spiritually and Physically -- if allowed to fester and pushed down, not acknowledged and released!

Our bodies talk to us -- What may start out as frustration, anger, hurt, and resentment can turn into illness and dis-ease in the physical body. Did you know that each organ and body part holds certain emotions?

As a child I fell and hurt myself many times, but that did not stop me from getting back up to walk or run again. However, I do remember being teased or told something hurtful and from that point on viewed myself in the light of the words that were spoken to me. It took YEARS to overcome and move past much of the hurt

5

experienced from those WORDS! Eventually, holding on to these words caused physical suffering also.

Most of us continue to hold onto emotional or mental hurt experienced from childhood, a relationship or some other traumatic events in our lives. As anyone who has been in an abusive relationship whether physical, mental or emotional (or any combination of them) can tell you, long after the wounds are healed, the emotional impact and scars may last for years!

I'm sure at some point you have experienced these emotions or situations:

• _Anger_ – It is not always a negative emotion, as humans we sometimes express our disappointment through anger. It can become an issue when it continues and begins to have a physical effect on us and/or when it becomes the "normal" way we deal with issues in our lives. Anger's physical response shows up in the form of increased heart rate, high blood pressure, headaches, adrenaline rush, problems with digestion, even as severe as a heart attack or stroke.

• _Sadness_ – We've all experienced sadness whether it is from a loss of a loved one, not getting something we've longed for, seeing something bad happen to another person. However, if you find yourself sad for prolonged periods of time, you may need to seek professional help or at least talk about your concerns to someone you trust and who supports you without criticizing your feelings. There's even a disorder called "SAD" – seasonal affective disorder which can occur during the winter months or in geographical areas where there is not a lot of sun over extended period of time. If this depression continues over an extended period of time, it may be suggested to take some type of supplementation or even use special lights that simulate the sun.

• _Grief_ – When we think of grief, it's normally in context of a loved one dying, however, it can also be experienced with the loss of a marriage, relationship, job, home, finances, material possessions, as well as loss of feeling of security such as a robbery or other

6

violations. Everyone handles grief differently and there is not set way that each person should deal with it.

There are several stages of grief including denial, guilt, anger, depression, bargaining, guilt and acceptances. They do not occur in any particular order and period of time. However, if a person finds it difficult to move forward in their lives due to a traumatic event, it is best to seek out some form of support to help begin to function better.

Other emotions include, fear, trauma (physical, emotional and mental), lack of confidence, hostility, heartache, worry, envy, and other unexpressed emotions.

Are you still holding on to any of them? Are they keeping you from moving forward or making good decisions in your life? If so, and you are having some type of physical ailments or problems — it's time to begin to LET GO — STARTING RIGHT NOW!!! It could save your life – literally!

It isn't always only the words that others say to us but also words we speak of, to and about ourselves. It's the little things said on a daily basis that add up and keep us "stuck". Did you know the subconscious mind cannot distinguish between what we think and what actually happens to us? If you think negative thoughts, you will draw negativity to you. So if you think positive, life-affirming thoughts, that also will be drawn to you.

During one of the most critical times when experiencing major health issues, I recall being in bed, barely able to speak above a whisper, unable to walk or do much for myself, I told a friend who was visiting at the time that one day I was going to get my naturopathic degree AND own a natural health store.

Of course, he did not believe me and thought that I was only making things worse by speaking on something that seemed impossible based on my condition at the time. He thought I was being unrealistic. My response to him was that if I did not see myself beyond where I was, I would always be there. Also, I believed that God had more in store for my life than the situation I was in at that particular time.

Was I being unrealistic and in denial about my condition at the time? No! I realized exactly what I was dealing with but also trusted that it would not be my destiny either. All I knew was that I was doing and would continue to do all that was within my power to improve my circumstances. When I spoke those words, I felt it in the depths of my SOUL, not just in my mind. I had no clue as to when or where or even HOW I was going to get the strength to accomplish my goals. But every day I did the best I could and kept as positive an attitude as I could.

It would be a few years later, but I did get my Bachelors of Natural Health and Masters/Doctorate in Naturopathy degrees. Eventually, I would own a natural health store! Sometimes even I forget the power of those words I spoke into the universe and prayed for years ago!

Consider these words or sayings that are contradictory to life:

• "I Love You to DEATH" try Loving me to LIFE!

• "No GOOD deed goes UNPUNISHED" – try No GOOD deed goes UNREWARDED!

According to the Attitudinal Awareness Guide by Ascension Mastery International (A.M.I.) "Healing ourselves requires that we remove the conditions that cause our dis-ease. In this process, we find that the causative factors of illness are not strictly physical problems. They can relate directly to the mental and emotional life we live as well.

Thoughts are neither good or bad. The unconscious mind accepts whatever you put into it. It does not judge whether it's right or wrong, negative or positive. It does not filter; it simply accepts it!

Our thoughts and feelings are powerful, dynamic forces that influence every aspect of our lives and are a major causative factor in either the health or dis-ease of our body and mind. How we feel and think about ourselves is what we become. Whether we realize it or not, our conscious and unconscious attitudes (belief systems) and feelings (emotions) powerfully affect the cells, tissues, and organs of our physical bodies, as well as the conditions we experience in the world around us."

Here are a few examples of how this works in different body parts:

- *Liver* -- Where resentment, suppressed anger and bitterness is held

- *Pancreas* -- Deals with the "sweetness" of life, loneliness and how one receives and give love

- *Joints* -- Deals with being flexible about life and situations – inability to "flow" with life circumstances and situations

- *Eyes* – Refusing to accept what we "see", what's in front of us or the truth

- *Back/Spine* – Worry about finances, carrying weight of too much responsibility, not having sufficient emotional support

- *Heart* – Associated with our desires (the desires of our hearts); expression or lack of expressing love (brokenhearted)

- *Skin* – Ability to let things go, surfacing of unexpressed emotions such as anger, resentment

- *Stomach* – Ability (or inability) to "digest" life's situations, critical and judgmental of self and others, not making wise choices in foods eaten

- *Uterus* – Feelings about one's femininity, motherhood and relationships with men

Holding on to the past (consciously or unconsciously) can be the *Weak Link* that is keeping you from healing your SOUL from diseases such as diabetes, cancer, high blood pressure, asthma, arthritis, back pain, joint pain, even sexually transmitted diseases.

This is not to say that you should blame yourself every time you develop an illness. This information is about making you aware of the connection between the physical, mental, emotional and spiritual aspects of health. It's about taking charge and controlling what you can in your life under all circumstances.

"Continuous modes of thinking and speaking produce body behaviors and postures and "eases" and "dis-eases". The person who has a permanently scowling face did not produce that by having joyous, loving thoughts…." Says Louise I. Hay, author of "You Can Heal Your Life". "Your thoughts about yourself, your situation, your life, and your body is reflected in, on and throughout your body."

What is the difference between emotional and mental health?

EMOTIONAL HEALTH – How do you deal with and respond to situations and issues in your life, your reactions to situations and how you recover from them.

MENTAL HEALTH – How you receive the information you get and how you process it in helping to make decisions about the situations, conditions that come your way.

There needs to be a balance between the two or you can express such issues as stress, anxiety, depression and other negative emotions. Imbalance in these areas can manifest in physical issues as well.

How do you know if you are balanced in these areas? Some indications can include:

- Being positive about life
- Awareness of your feelings

10

- Knowing when you have reached your limit and need assistance in resolving your problems
- Your priorities are in order
- You are happy with your life
- Your stress levels are low
- You have healthy relationships in all areas of your life

To help balance your life try the following:

- Meditate
- Get some "ME" time (spend and set aside time with yourself)
- Eat healthy
- Read books on your favorite subjects
- Have a hobby
- Spend quality time with friends and family
- Volunteer (helping others can increase your self-esteem and helps you not to concentrate so much on what's not going well in your life, also makes you appreciate your blessings which can sometimes appear as problematic)

Understanding how the mental and emotional parts of us are not harmonized, ultimately, the physical body will begin to reflect the imbalance. Striving to keep all aspects of what comprises your SOUL, is a constant work in progress.

LINK #2

LET ME HEAR YOUR BODY TALK!:
YOUR BODY SYSTEMS

"Even so the body is not made up of one part but of many. Now if the foot should say, "Because I am not a hand, I do not belong to the body," it would not for that reason stop being part of the body. And if the ear should say, "Because I am not an eye, I do not belong to the body," it would not for that reason stop being part of the body.

If the whole body were an eye, where would the sense of hearing be? If the whole body were an ear, where would the sense of smell be? But in fact God has placed the parts in the body, every one of them, just as he wanted them to be. If they were all one part, where would the body be? As it is, there are many parts, but one body.

The eye cannot say to the hand, "I don't need you!" And the head cannot say to the feet, "I don't need you!" On the contrary, those parts of the body that seem to be weaker are indispensable, and the parts that we think are less honorable we treat with special honor. And the parts that are unpresentable are treated with special modesty, while our presentable parts need no special treatment.

But God has put the body together, giving greater honor to the parts that lacked it, so that there should be no division in the body, but that its parts should have equal concern for each other. If one part suffers, every part suffers with it; if one part is honored, every part rejoices with it."

1 Corinthians 12:14-26

These verses confirm that each part of the body and each body system does not work in isolation, but together. Each system has very specific functions and some overlap with other systems to ensure maximum overall health benefits to the body as a whole. Just as these systems overlap and interact to keep the body *healthy,* when out of balance, can also *cause* problems in several systems.

We are the sum total of ALL our parts, not just the physical but the emotional, mental and spiritual parts of our total being. When one organ, system or body part is distress, it can affect many other parts of the body, mind and spirit.

By taking a brief review of the body systems and the organs associated with them to get an understanding of the organs and systems inside of us, how each functions and you will get an idea of what causes imbalances in our bodies and how these imbalances effect our health. This isn't meant to be a biology lesson but simply to refresh your memory on some of the many "jobs" the body performs that allow us to live healthfully on a daily basis.

I have listed the different body systems and a little bit about how they function to give you some insight into the importance of keeping the body and the sum of its part intact.

DIGESTIVE/INTESTINAL –This system ensures proper ingestion, digestion, and assimilation of nutrients and elimination of waste from the body. Some say that digestion actually starts with the eyes – LOOKING at something that we would like to eat causes us to salivate. However, the physical process of digestion starts in the mouth, beginning with the first bite when saliva is secreted to help break down food with enzymes as well as lubricate and moisturize food so that we can swallow easily and comfortably.

The tongue not only helps move food around in the mouth but is where the many taste buds exist which allow us to taste sweet, sour, salty, bitter and sweet. As this pre-digested food goes down the esophagus – which is only about 10 inches long and about 1 inch in diameter, through a reflex action, food travels to the stomach.

In the stomach, acids and enzymes are waiting and prepared to break down foods even further. This substance then travels to the small intestines where nutrients are absorbed and goes into the bloodstream. The portion that does not contain nutrients are separated and called wastes. These wastes, including any fiber, is then moved into the colon to be passed as bowel movement.

Digestion requires more energy than any other process in the body. Notice how tired and sleepy you become after eating a large or wrongly combined meal? Blood rushes to the stomach to help process the food eaten.

The organs that are part of the *digestive/intestinal* systems include:

Primary Organs
- Mouth
- Stomach
- Pharynx
- Esophagus
- Small Intestine
- Large Intestines

Accessory Organs
- Teeth
- Salivary Glands
- Tongue
- Liver
- Gallbladder
- Pancreas
- Rectum
- Anal Canal
- Appendix

When any of these organs are out of balance - Think: constipation, gas, acid reflux, heartburn, diabetes, gallstones, diarrhea, dental and gum issues, difficulty swallowing, irritable bowel syndrome, Chrohn's disease, colitis, sore throat.

GLANDULAR

Reproductive — In order for reproduction to take place, a woman has to be able to produce eggs for fertilization which initially involves having her menstrual cycle. This involves the body preparing for the possibility of pregnancy. If does not occur, the lining of the uterus which contains the unfertilized egg(s) and blood sheds. This process is repeated monthly until and unless pregnancy occurs.

In addition to reproduction, this system is responsible for the development of hormones which allow sexual characteristic development. These hormones include estrogen, progesterone, follicle stimulating hormone (FSH) and luteinizing hormone.

This system consists of:

WOMEN
- Ovaries
- Fallopian Tubes
- Uterus
- Vagina
- Vulva
- Breasts

When any of these organs are out of balance - Think: infertility, PMS, vaginal yeast infections, menopause, fibroids, fibrocystic breast, breast cancer, ovarian and endometrial cancers, STD's (sexually transmitted disease), PID (pelvic inflammatory disease), frigidity.

MEN
Reproductive — In order for a woman's egg to be fertilized it must be joined with sperm.

The male hormones are:
- Testes
- Prostate
- Vas Deferens

- Penis
- Urethra
- Scrotum

When any of these organs are out of balance – Think: prostate and testicular cancer, low sperm count, impotence, erectile dysfunction, STD's (sexually transmitted disease)

Endocrine — This specialized system of glands produces and releases hormones into the blood directly. Similar to the nervous system except it functions in a slower, longer lasting way. These glands have an effect on every organ, cell and body function in the body.

This system consists of:
- Pancreas
- Ovaries
- Testes
- Pituitary
- Pineal
- Hypothalamus
- Thyroid
- Parathyroid
- Thymus
- Adrenals

When any of these organs are out of balance - Think: Obesity, Adrenal fatigue, chronic fatigue syndrome, Type 1 and Type 2 diabetes, metabolic disorders, growth disorders

CARDIOVASCULAR/CIRCULATORY – The main function is that of transporting oxygen and carbon dioxide, hormones, nutrients as well as cellular by-products (waste) to be released from the body.

This system consists of:
- Heart
- Blood Vessels

- Arteries
- Veins
- Capillaries

When these organs are out of balance - Think: High Blood Pressure, heart attacks, angina, strokes, blood clots, arteriosclerosis, atherosclerosis, etc.

<u>NERVOUS</u> - This system is responsible for control and integration of body functions, including communication between body functions and recognition of sensations inside (internal stimulus) and outside (external stimulus) of the body. It consists of two parts: the central nervous system and the peripheral nervous system which includes autonomic nervous system.

The central nervous system takes information it receives and sends it out to all parts of the body to coordinate its various activities.

The *peripheral nervous system* connects the nerves between the brain and spinal cord together. These nerves relate to the surface of the skin as well as skeletal muscles. As part of the peripheral nervous system, the autonomic nervous system regulates those functions of the body that occur without our conscious control such as heart rate, glandular secretions, stomach contractions, intestinal tract. It is our "fight" or "flight, "rest and digest" and "feed and greed" stimulator.

The *autonomic nervous system* consists of 2 distinct systems: the sympathetic nervous system and the parasympathetic nervous system.

The *sympathetic nervous system* is your "fight" or "flight" stimulator and deals with those actions that happen without being conscious of them such as heartbeat, digestion, respiration, kidney function, adrenals.

For example, if you're driving along the road and everything is flowing just fine, then suddenly, someone cuts you off in traffic, immediately your heartrate will increase, your stomach may feel twisted in a knot, your blood pressure goes up. You become angry or scared. You may start cussing, blowing your horn and some may even want to get out of their car, want to cause the other person some type of physical harm OR they may choose to get away from that situation as soon as possible. In either case, the body has a physical reaction to what's happening.

The *parasympathetic nervous system* is the body's "rest and digest" and "feed and breed" stimulator. It deals with activities that happen when the body is at rest, particularly after rest, such as digestion, bowel movements, urination, sensations, even sexual arousal.

This system consists of:
- Brain
- Spinal Cord
- Nerves

When the nervous system is out of balance -- Think: Multiple Sclerosis, Parkinson disease, strokes, brain tumors, brain cancer, Tourette's syndrome, Alzheimer's, dementia, (now you can see how this system imbalance can cause the severe symptoms of these diseases!)

RESPIRATORY – Permits the movement of air into the alveoli (tiny, thin-walled sacs) of the lungs. It goes without saying that going even a few minutes without oxygen is NOT a good thing! Not only do we need to breathe in oxygen, we must get rid of carbon dioxide by breathing out. This constant intake of oxygen and release of carbon dioxide is what allows our cells to function properly.

This system consists of:
- Mouth
- Nose
- Trachea
- Tonsils

18

- Pharynx
- Larynx
- Lungs
- Diaphragm

When any of these organs are out of balance -- Think: asthma, bronchitis, emphysema, sinusitis, tonsillitis, sore throat, flu, pulmonary embolism, lung cancer

LYMPHATIC/IMMUNE – Responsible for the movement of nutrients that are fat-related and fluids, particularly large molecules from spaces of tissues around cells.

This system, simply put, is your first line of defense against, microorganisms, germs, bacteria. Fungus, viruses, parasites, tumors and toxins inside and outside of the body. It helps the body get rid of unwanted toxins, debris including dead cells internally and fights off dangerous substances from entering the body. *The body contains more lymphatic fluid than it does blood.*

This system consists of:
- Lymph nodes
- Spleen
- Lymph vessels
- Bronchi
- Thymus
- Bone marrow

When any of these organs are out of balance -- Think: Cancer, edema, viruses, infections, allergies, boils, autoimmune disorders.

URINARY/EXCRETORY -- Cleans poisonous waste products from the blood, maintains water, electrolyte and acid-balance in the body. The urinary system, specifically – the kidneys -- is critical to maintaining fluid homeostasis (or balance) in the body.

This system consists of:
- Kidneys

- Urinary Bladder
- Ureters

When any of these organs are out of balance - Think: bladder *infections, nephritis, kidney stones, gout, renal disease, high blood pressure.*

STRUCTURAL

Skeletal – Provides a rigid frame for the body that provides support and protection. The joints of this system allows the body parts to move.
This system consists of:
- Bones
- Joints

When any of these organs are out of balance - Think: arthritis, rheumatoid arthritis, osteoporosis, carpal tunnel syndrome, lupus.

Muscular – Besides allowing movement and maintaining body posture, they are responsible for maintaining a constant core body temperature.

This system consists of the following muscles:
- *Voluntary (skeletal)* – These muscles allow body movement and include biceps, triceps, gluteal, abdominal, deltoids (shoulder), and pectoral (chest), muscles.
- *Involuntary (smooth)* – These are muscles controlled unconsciously through the brain and body. The uterus, esophagus, bladder, muscles behind the eyes, stomach, intestines are examples of involuntary muscles.
- *Cardiac (heart)* – These muscles are mainly in the heart and similarly like involuntary muscles, cannot be consciously controlled. These muscles are self-stimulating for the most part.

When any of these organs are out of balance - Think: fibromyalgia, muscular dystrophy, myasthenia gravis, cardiomyopathy (weakened heart muscle), myocarditis (inflammation of heart muscle).

INTEGUMENTARY – The body's primary source of protection (mainly the skin) against outside elements as well as regulating body temperature through sweating, and operates as a sense organ.

This system consists of:
- Skin
- Nails
- Hairs
- Sense Receptors
- Sweat glands
- Oil glands

When any of these organs are out of balance - Think: premature baldness, alopecia, eczema, psoriasis, dry or oil skin.

As you can see, if any one of these systems is out of balance, illness and dis-ease can easily become apparent. When we think of different body parts and systems, it is usually in the context of them working independently. However, most systems work inter-dependently of another and/or perform similar functions. Therefore, when it comes to dis-ease, illness as well as health, it is not possible to completely isolate body parts, organs and systems to keep the body in balance.

For example, experiencing a headache may not simply be related to the head and circulation. Problems associated with headaches can be as simple as sniffing something that doesn't agree with you and causes discomfort to something as serious as a stroke or worst.

Some headaches may stem from imbalances in the nervous system, but can also be caused by constipation which is associated with the digestive/intestinal systems. This can be the result of not drinking enough water, sluggish liver, lack of sufficient fiber in the diet, even allergies. When this occurs toxins build up in the body and have no escape through the normal eliminative channels and can result in a headache. Once the problem is corrected, the symptoms may disappear.

LINK #3

ARE YOU MY TYPE? :
FINDING YOUR BODY TYPE

How does body *type* affect health? As humans we have the same body *systems*, however, our bodies are not all shaped the same (variety is the spice of life!). Our body "types" can potentially have different effects on health -- positively or negatively.

What does your body type have to do with your health? Well, a lot more than you realize. Your body type can affect your chances of developing certain diseases, the types of foods you eat, the best exercises for your body type, even to what clothes look best on you!

Now let's take a look at each of these body types and see how closely you may fit a particular body type. *NOTE: not everyone will fit in any or all of these categories and none of these are absolute characteristics of any one person or body type.*

What are considered basic body types and which one or combinations come closest to your body type. There are as many as 25 different body types, but we will focus on the 4 basic types for women and the 3 basic types for men.

WOMEN

For women they are *APPLE, PEAR, BANANA and HOURGLASS* body shapes.

APPLE
BODY SHAPE
- Narrow hips and pelvis
- Weight gain tends to be in abdominal and upper part of body
- Stores fat in the stomach and chest area

- Has to work harder at keeping waistline trim
- Tendency toward producing more male hormones than other body types
- Tends to have cellulite in trunk, abdominal and upper buttocks areas
- Anabolic (increase build-up of muscles) metabolism
- May have shapely legs and bottom
- Athletic build

HEALTH BENEFITS/RISKS
- More at risk of developing cardiac issues and hypertension, diabetes and high cholesterol
- Prominent mental and physical strength
- Tend to gain and lose weight quickly

DIET
- Foods should include low glycemic such as fresh fruits and vegetables, nuts, seeds; unsaturated fats such as salmon, lentils, whole grain breads); lean meats

EXERCISE
- Cardio exercises work best (pushups, sit-ups, abdominal curls, jogging, walking, aerobics)

STYLE OF CLOTHES
- Wearing looser tops and dresses can make the waist appear slimmer

BANANA
BODY SHAPE
- Long-limbed with fine and narrow bones
- No problem maintaining weight/difficulty gaining weight
- High metabolic rate
- May not develop cellulite, but if so, will be on buttocks and back of thighs
- Athletic

- Weight gain is usually centered in stomach area

HEALTH BENEFITS/RISKS
- Usually don't have to be concerned about weight gain unless they don't take care of their health.

DIET
- Tends to like unhealthy substances such as caffeine, nicotine, artificial sweeteners, etc. without many obvious side effects
- As with most body types, processed foods should be avoided,
- Sugar should also be greatly reduced or avoided
- Proteins such as nuts, eggs, lean meat should be included in diet
- Whole grains, brown rice, quinoa, amaranth should be included in the diet as well
- Fresh vegetables such as leafy greens should also be included

EXERCISE
- By toning the upper and lower parts of the body, can develop a more curvaceous appearing physique.
- Exercises such as boxing, weight lifting and swimming can help build upper body
- Exercises such as squats, lunges and leg raises can develop lower body.
- For maintenance of the heart and improvement of circulation of the blood, it is recommended to do cardio at least 30 minutes a day.

STYLE OF CLOTHES
- Belts
- Dresses/skirts that flair out can add curve appeal
- Frilly and lacy dresses/skirts also can add definition to the banana shaped figure
- Does not gain fat in the body quickly (unless eating an unhealthy diet)

PEAR

BODY TYPE

- One of the most common body types for men and women
- Lower half of body larger than top, especially in hips and thighs
- Small waist
- Estrogen-dominant
- More fat around thighs, hips and buttocks with cellulite
- Will lose weight in upper part of body but not from buttocks when on low-fat diet

HEALTH BENEFITS/RISKS

- Issues of concern are eating disorders such as bulimia and anorexia, osteoporosis and varicose veins
- Less likely to develop heart disease and diabetes due to lack of visceral fat which is a type of fat that is stored in the stomach region and can potentially have an effect on hormone function.

DIET

- Avoid foods that are high on the glycemic index such as sugars, processed foods
- Stick to low glycemic foods such as whole grains, leafy green vegetables, fruits such apples, berries. Grapefruit
- May crave fat and sugar

EXERCISE

- Aerobic exercise and strength training are ideal for this body type
- Forty-five minutes of cardio 3-4 times a week will help ward off fat deposits

STYLE OF CLOTHES

- Clothes that emphasize the top of the body work best such as puffy sleeves, cowl necks, push up bras
- Avoid tight fitting jeans or pants that bring more attention to the bottom half
- Wearing darker clothes on bottom half also work
- Heels are a good way to look slimmer

HOURGLASS
BODY TYPE

- Tends to store fat in stomach, buttocks, thighs and upper arms
- Gain and lose weight quickly
- Joints (knees, ankles, spine) are more susceptible to pain
- Represents femininity, youth and fertility
- Desired most by men in almost all cultures
- Well balanced at top and bottom with small waist

HEALTH BENEFITS/RISKS

- The fat that is stored in the hip area is beneficial due to its hormone levels
- Tend to have less complications during childbirth
- Can gain weight in waistline if not taken care of and become susceptible to Type 2 diabetes and other health issues

DIET

- Should avoid high glycemic foods such as white foods such as white flour, potatoes, rice as well as processed foods, bananas.
- Also avoid highly saturated fats such as fried foods, ice cream, milkshakes and other junk foods
- Incorporate healthy fats such as flax oil, extra virgin olive oil (preferably organic), coconut oil, raw nuts
- Calcium and Vitamin D3 for joint health

EXERCISE

- Best exercises include bicep curls, sit ups, squats, Pilates, yoga, jogging, cycling and aerobic exercise

STYLE OF CLOTHES

- Wide belts that accentuate the waistline
- Pencil skirts, A-line dresses
- Jackets that are fitted
- V-neck tops

MEN

The basic body types are ECTOMORPH (Thyroid), Android/
MESOMORPH, and Lymphatic/ENDOMORPH.

ECTOMORPH (THYROID)
BODY TYPE
- Light frame and build
- Have difficulty gaining weight
- Struggles to build muscle
- Metabolism is fast
- Small shoulders
- Flat chest
- Very easily loses fat

DIET
- May need additional calories to maintain or gain weight due to their fast metabolism
- Need to include high protein sources to help build muscle mass
- May have to use supplements to help increase muscle mass
- Still does not mean you should eat junk food (empty calories) to put on weight. Eat a well-balanced diet, i.e. 50% healthy carbohydrates, 30% protein and 20% good fats.

EXERCISE
- Although cardio exercise is great for heart health, should keep down to about 30 minutes a day so as not to lose muscle

MESOMORPH (ANDROID)
BODY TYPE
- Large bone structure
- Strong muscle definition
- Easily gains and maintains muscle
- Loses and gains weight quite easily
- Broad shoulders and chest
- Thin waistline

DIET

- Two of the most important nutrients are protein (lean and fat free) for the muscles and calcium for bone and joint health

EXERCISE

- Recommend bench presses, squats, deadlifts, dumbbell flies, leg extensions and lunges to maintain physique
- Cardio exercises can be included but not necessarily a high amount due to the other exercises, if done on regular basis

ENDOMORPH (LYMPHATIC)
BODY TYPE

- Easily gains weight
- Hard to lose fat
- Slow metabolism
- Not very well defined muscles
- Short build
- Thick legs and arms
- Strong, muscular upper legs
- Tend to be "rounder" shaped
- Broad but not muscular shoulders

DIET

- Should limit carbohydrate intake and avoid junk food
- Carbohydrates to include should be unrefined and whole grains
- Avoid refined carbohydrates
- Eat 5-6 meals a day to keep up metabolic rate
- Increase fruits and vegetables

EXERCISE

- Change up exercise routine to avoid muscle fatigue
- Can build muscle faster when training on a regular basis (about 5 days/week)
- Cardio exercises are important such as walking, jogging and cycling
- Weight training using moderate weights and around 10

repetitions

It's important to remember that we can't change our height, bone structure and basic body shape. It IS important that we understand how all of these factors affect our health and well-being – either positively or negatively – and learn to EMBRACE our beauty, not by society's ideals but what make us the unique individuals God made us!

As mentioned before, your body type can change due to lack of exercise, diet, illness and other factors. If you are interested in changing or improving your body type, look at the body type you most fit and make changes to your diet, do specific exercises that may improve specific areas of the body.

LINK #4

CLEAN UP YOUR ACT!:
DETOXING AND CLEANSING

These two words have been overused and misunderstood since the recent "holistic health" explosion over the past 15-20 years. I'm often asked "how do I detox my body" or "I'm doing a detox, but I don't see anything happening".

Well, first of all let me say that there are probably as many different types of detoxes and cleansings as there probably are people on the face of the earth!! -- Maybe a slight exaggeration there!! ☺ But the truth of the matter is one must first understand the WHY, then WHAT, WHEN AND HOW of cleansing and detoxing.

WHY – The reason you want to do a detox or cleanse is the first question that needs to be addressed. Are you doing it because it's the popular thing to do? Are you doing it because your friend, family member, co-worker, etc. tried it and it worked well for them? Do you want to lose weight? Start a better lifestyle? All of these questions and more need to be considered.

WHAT – What are you attempting to accomplish? This question overlaps with the "why" in that you need to consider what the end result will be. Is it just a starting point to achieve maximum health? What specific organs or body systems will you be targeting? Is there a specific health issue you want to address? What efforts will it take to begin, complete and finish the program?

HOW – Another very important question! How will you go about instituting the program? Will you accomplish it by using herbal supplements? Juicing? Fruits and Vegetables? Organ specific programs (programs focusing on specific organs such as liver, kidney, colon, etc.)? Seasonal detoxes? Food elimination? Detox pads? Some form of bodywork (massage, reflexology, acupuncture)?

There are so many options, however, I will focus only on a couple that I have used periodically and successfully. One is a Liver Cleanse and the other works to rid the body of excess mucous called "The Master Cleanse" or the "Lemonade Diet". Both have been used to lose weight.

THE LIVE-R – IF THE LIVER FAILS, THE BODY DIES
LIVER HEALTH AND WELLNESS

Every organ in the body is important and has its role to play, however, the liver has to perform more functions than any other organ. I wanted to include a chapter specifically on the liver because it is often overlooked in respect to many of the degenerative diseases wreaking havoc on so many people today.

Even when the diet and digestion is good, if the liver is unable to perform its over 500 jobs properly, the cells of the body will be grossly malnourished. It's not just what we eat and digest, but how well the liver utilizes and transforms food nutrients into forms the bloodstream can transport to the body's cells, and the cells can use to perform its functions.

The liver is the body's LARGEST INTERNAL organ, weighing three to five pounds in adults. The liver is the master organ for creating optimal nutrition for the 50 trillion cells in your body. It uses 12 – 20% of the body's total energy, and it must generate this energy to its own cells. Now that's a LOT of work for just one organ! Whew!

The liver routinely performs over 500 known functions to regulate your cell's metabolism. It transforms toxins into harmless chemicals for excretion, and digestively absorbed nutrients into the proper biochemical forms your cells can use to function. Yet the liver is probably the organ most assaulted by toxic modern lifestyles, full of pollution, stress, junk foods, drugs, etc.

Research has shown that in the US over 40,000 deaths a year are due to liver disease. Yet most people will never suffer from hepatitis, cirrhosis, or jaundice -- the "classic" liver diseases. Toxic modern lifestyles may however promote what's considered "subclinical" or secondary liver dysfunction.

Effects of toxic liver and gallbladder include:

- Diabetes
- Hypoglycemia
- Thyroid problems
- Heart Disease
- High cholesterol
- Cirrhosis
- Hormonal imbalances
- Constipation
- Flatulence (excessive gas)
- Indigestion
- Jaundice
- Alcoholism
- Drug addiction
- Chrohn's disease
- Nausea
- Lupus
- Coagulation (blood clotting factors)

Only a few of these dis-eases are directly associated with the liver. However, each of them has some correlation to the many functions of the liver. For example, did you know that the hormones T3 and T4 are necessary for good thyroid function and are manufactured in the liver? So if the liver is sluggish and unable to operate at its highest capacity, proper metabolism is disrupted.

Even though our cells die and replace themselves, the liver is the only organ that regenerates itself. If the liver is damaged and part of it removed, it will actually grow back to its normal size fairly quickly, unlike other body parts. Now how amazing is that?!

Food Choices That Improve Liver Health

The foods we eat and how we take care of ourselves greatly affects how our liver works. It is important to choose foods that will help keep your liver healthy. Good nutrition can also help to rebuild the liver and replace damaged liver cells. It can also help the liver form new cells.

There are many foods that can help the liver remain healthy as well as rebuild it if damaged. The foods listed below are used to help to detoxify and to rebuild the liver.

Oils – Flaxseed (linseed), extra virgin olive oil, peanut safflower, sunflower

Spices – Basil, cayenne, cinnamon, cloves, coriander, cumin, dill, fennel, garlic, ginger, oregano, nutmeg, rosemary, sage, turmeric

Vegetables – Cruciferous vegetables such as broccoli, Brussels sprouts, cabbage, cauliflower; as well as asparagus, beets, carrots, collards, cucumbers, kale, parsley, spinach, tomatoes, zucchini

Fruits – Apples, avocado, Berries (blueberries, blackberries, cranberries, raspberries, strawberries,), lemons, melons, peaches

Whenever possible choose organic, however, do not let this keep you from eating plenty of fresh fruits and vegetables as well as incorporating liver-enriching spices and oils in the diet.

When choosing a diet that is good for the liver it is important to think of fresh fruits and vegetables. You will want to eat plenty of dark green, leafy vegetables and colored fruits. These foods contain enzymes, fiber, vitamins, antibiotic substances, and nutrients to help fight cancer.

Included in maintaining a good diet to help the liver, don't forget the importance of water. Ideally, you should drink ½ your body's weight in ounces of water per day (ex. A person weighing 160 lbs. should drink 80 oz. water/day). Water helps to get rid of the toxins that the liver has broken down and removes it from the body. (We will discuss water more in an upcoming chapter.)

Even when doing everything you can within your power to stay healthy, the everyday course of life can still put a strain on the liver. Just breathing in toxins from the outdoor air from car exhausts, chemicals we use in the house, and on our bodies cause the liver to work harder and harder to detoxify and eliminate toxins. Not to mention the many jobs it has including the following:

- Manufacturing bile salts that help break down fats which also help in proper elimination

- Helping to break down hormones such as insulin, estrogen, adrenaline and other hormones

- Producing cholesterol into forms that the body can use effectively

- Storing nutrients such as iron, Vitamins A, D and B12 to be released when the body is in need of them.

These are just a few of the functions of the liver. It was important for me to include the liver functions over all the other organs in the body because as stated in the headline of this section – *"IF THE LIVER FAILS – THE BODY DIES!!"* Yes, it's true if the heart, brain and other vital organs die, you will also die. However, so many diseases can also start because the liver is not functioning at full capacity. Paying attention to this organ's function or malfunction can affect so many other body systems.

LIVER/GALLBLADDER CLEANSE

With all the health issues I was experiencing, it took a while to recognize how out of balance my liver had become. It wasn't until I was in my mid-forties (while going through that lovely "change of life", did I realized that many of the hormonal issues I was going through, stemmed from having a "fatty" liver. I gained 40 pounds over a 4-year period. No matter how much I changed and adjusted my diet, I couldn't stop the weight gain. I decided to cleanse my liver and after about 9 months, I lost 30 of those 40 pounds.

Doing a liver/gallbladder cleanse is one of the single MOST powerful ways to jumpstart your body in a short period of time! Another job of the liver is to make bile – 1 to 1.5 quarts in a day! The liver is full of tubes (biliary tubing) that deliver bile to one large tube (the common bile duct). The gallbladder is attached to the common bile duct and acts as a storage reservoir. When you eat fats, it triggers the gallbladder to empty itself after about 20 minutes, and the bile that is stored continues down the common bile duct to the intestine.

At this point the liver should have removed most of the toxins (at least those it recognizes). Bile is used to remove heavy metals (cadmium, copper, lead, mercury, radioactive elements, and more) from the body as well as other toxins. But, depending upon how the liver is functioning, it may cause those toxins to come back inside of the body.

The liver is producing bile from cholesterol by converting it into bile acids. Bile also contains a lot of toxins that have to be removed from the body. But the problem is that bile is going directly into our intestines, and by doing this we have a chance of absorbing those toxins again into the bloodstream.

There are several ways to cleanse the liver such as with herbs, other cleanses and foods (which are mentioned later). Here's a liver cleansing regimen I have used periodically over the years and found I have a "better attitude" and feeling better in general when doing so.

NOTE: Do not do a liver cleanse or any other detox program without consulting your health care professional. CHECK WITH YOUR HEALTH CARE PROFESSIONAL BEFORE TRYING THIS CLEANSE IF YOU ARE ALREADY EXPERIENCING LIVER OR GALLBLADDER PROBLEMS OR ARE ON MEDICATIONS.

This formula is not for the fainthearted and sometimes it is best to prepare the body a few days or a week prior to performing this cleanse. Approximately a week prior to doing this cleanse it is suggested that you adjust your eating habits such as eliminating all fried foods, greatly reduce refined and processes foods, increase fresh fruits, raw and/or light steamed vegetables. Eat a fairly "clean" diet, this will help to prevent experiencing the effects of detoxing as the liver releases old wastes and toxins into the bloodstream. This "health crisis" may cause nausea or vomiting.

Instructions for Liver Cleanse

(repeat process three nights in a row)

In separate glasses (you can also mix the lemon juice and olive in 1 cup if desired) pour the following:

4 OZ. EXTRA VIRGIN OLIVE OIL -- Acts as "fresh" oil flushing out the old oil (bile, cholesterol, toxins, poisons that have accumulated over time). Look at this as you would your car's engine. To keep your car's engine functioning at its highest capacity you must change the oil about every 3 months or 3,000 miles.

We sometimes take better care of our cars than we take care of our bodies. Would you continue to drive your car for years at a time without changing the oil and filter? Of course not, unless you are willing to risk ruining the engine and as you may know, that can be quite expensive.

Isn't YOUR engine (body) worth preserving and keeping lubricated and running in top condition? What good is a well-tuned, smooth running vehicle if you find yourself in a position where you are unable to function properly? Yet we assault our bodies on a daily basis.

4 OZ. FRESH SQUEEZED LEMON JUICE (ABOUT 4-5 LEMONS depending on size and freshness) -- Acts as an astringent to loosen up mucous that has accumulated in the body. Although lemons are considered an acid fruit, it becomes alkaline in the body.

8 OZ. SPRING WATER -- helps to flush out the toxins and "slug" that the oil and lemon juice have loosened up and helps remove them from the liver and gallbladder.

- Drink in the above order right before bedtime. Make this the last thing done before going to bed.

- Then lie on RIGHT side with a pillow under right side for about 20 minutes and repeat 3 nights in a row. This puts pressure on the liver to activate the cleanse. You do not have to stay in this position all night!

- Ideally, the next morning there should have been some bowel movement. You may notice in the stool, for lack of a better term, wrinkled sweet peas or raisins. These are gallstones.* YES, you must LOOK ◔◔ to see what your stool looks like!

Results will vary with each individual. This is just a typical scenario. Even if there are no obvious gallstones, it does not mean that you are not obtaining desired outcome.

THE MASTER CLEANSE or LEMONADE DIET

Another cleanse I have used with great results is the "Master or "Lemonade" Cleanse. When I initially tried this cleanse I was not able to complete more than 1 day before I felt bad. At the time I was still having severe blood sugar issues. My blood sugar would drop too fast and I would feel awful. I did not attempt it again for at least another 10 years! Eventually, I was able to do 3 days with ease. Then I did several 10 day cleanses and felt very good while on them. Then I finally did a 28-day cleanse! It was definitely a challenge but I felt pretty good on it. Of course, I lost, on average, about a pound a day.

I believe I was successful on the 10 and 28 day cleanses because I mentally prepared myself each time and planned far enough in advance (about 2-3 weeks) before I did them. I also read _"The_

Complete Master Cleanse, A Step by Step Guide to the Lemonade Diet" by Tom Woloshyn. To be successful, he states "Some people like to prepare their body before a cleanse. They go on a vegetarian diet for four or five days before starting the cleanse, ramping up to an all-veggie diet before starting the cleanse itself. This simpler diet will be less stressful on the body and will help with the eventual elimination of some of your poor food choices. Eating such a diet will make it easier for you to transition to the Master Cleanse."

Some of the benefits include, improved sleep, fewer allergy problems, clearer skin, reduction of addiction dependence, and of course, weight loss.

Each time I decided to do this cleanse, I read his book from cover to cover. What I found learned more and more about how to successfully complete the cleanse. However, I noticed that shortly after completing the 10 day sessions, I would get flu-like symptoms and for the first time developed bronchitis. Part of the problem was adjusting to the climate in Tennessee. However, I also realized my body had reached the point where it was beginning to get used to eliminating toxins and I stopped! My body had adjusted to the detox process and continued to throw off toxins in the form of mucous and it became overwhelmed.

After I completed the 28-day cleanse, I noticed these symptoms did not appear. This length of time allowed my body to really release while still on the cleanse. People have been known to stay on this cleanse nearly a year and their bodies reached a point where their weight settled to a point on the scale that was naturally comfortable for them. I do not suggest anyone does a cleanse that length without the strict supervision of a health care professional who is experienced in monitoring someone on a cleanse or detox program.

Both programs can be used periodically but not together. It's best to spread out the time that you do them so that you do not overtax the liver and allow your body to adjust to the transition your body goes through on each program.

LINK #5

THE "STUFF" WE'RE MADE OF: VITAMINS, MINERALS AND BASIC NUTRIENTS

What composes the wondrous machine called the human body? What makes up our cells, body parts, and organs? Just as the earth is composed of almost 75% water, so is the human body. Both contain minerals that are essential for existence. (Ashes to ashes, dust to dust). Vitamins are mainly produced in the body.

Because of the depletion of minerals in the ground, most of us are more mineral deficient than vitamin deficient.

What is the role of vitamins, minerals and other nutrients in the body?

Our bodies are miraculous in its ability to perform and almost infinite number of functions. It is important that we nourish it with the correct nutrients so that it can perform for a long period of time. Even when we do not treat it so well, it will continue, in spite of us, to work and function at its best and it is so forgiving that if we go back to eating well and taking care of it, it can often times repair itself to its previous state of wellness.

In order for the body to function at its fullest capacity it is essential to 1) provide it with good nutrition, 2) have a sufficient amount of food, 3) you must eat the RIGHT foods, and 4) eat them in the correct proportions.

This is where vitamins, minerals and other basic nutrients come in. We all know that most foods, meaning **natural, whole** foods, contain some of these elements. The amount depends on the source of food. These sources have certain types of vitamins, minerals and other nutrients that are a part of a balanced diet.

VITAMINS -- There are 2 types of vitamins: fat soluble and water soluble.

Fat soluble which is not soluble in water, but is in fat, is stored in the body and when taken in large doses will be stored in the body over long periods of time, can become toxic (except vitamin E). It takes some time to recognize when there is a deficiency in these vitamins; they are absorbed through the intestines in the same manner as fat. Because they are stored mainly in the liver, an adequate supply can last for months at a time.

Examples of fat soluble vitamins include:
Vitamin A (Retinol and Carotenes) – Known mainly for its effect on improving vision. It also helps to destroy free radicals, metabolizes carbohydrates in the liver, aids in the development and growth of bones. It is necessary in excellent hearing, smell and taste.

It is high in beta-carotene (a non-toxic antioxidant) which can be found in carrots, pumpkin, sweet potatoes, apricots and cantaloupe, leafy green vegetables and some dairy products like milk, egg yolks and cheese.

Deficiencies appear as:
- poor night vision
- problems with teeth such as loss of enamel on teeth and increased cavities
- more likely to have infection, particularly in the respiratory tract
- Wounds tend to heal slower

Vitamin D – the body produces this vitamin through direct sunlight. It is also important in the development of bones and building up the immune system. Needed to properly absorb phosphorus and calcium from the intestines as well as keeping proper blood levels of these minerals.

FOOD SOURCES:
- egg yolk

- fish
- fish oils
- cereals

Deficiencies appear as:
- Osteoporosis
- Weak and soft bones

Vitamin E – As an antioxidant, this vitamin helps vitamins A and C and EFAs (essential fatty acids) from being destroyed. Can protect the cardiovascular system. Keeps red blood cells from being destroyed, is part of the natural process of reproduction by helping prevent recurrent miscarriage, may be useful in helping with leg cramps and helps slow down aging.

Vitamin E can be found in nut seeds, grains and vegetable oils.

Deficiencies appear as:
- Generally, not a problem because it is found in most foods
- May sometimes be found in premature babies
- Persons with issues with fat absorption over an extended period of time

Vitamin K – Helps with the coagulation of blood and a deficiency can lead to bleeding risks. It is produced by intestinal bacteria and is part of the formation of bones and cell growth.

Sources of this vitamin appear in dark, leafy green vegetables, the outer leaves of cabbage (the greenest parts), peas, cauliflower.

Deficiency appears as:
- Because a newborn's intestine lack bacteria when they are born, generally it is recommended they get a dosage of Vitamin K right after birth.
- Adults with vitamin K deficiency is usually due to an issue of malabsorption such as in the case of diarrhea, obstruction of the bile duct or from certain medications.

Water soluble are not soluble in fat, but in water. Because it is not stored in the body, these vitamins must be replaced daily; storage, heat and cooking destroy these vitamins quickly. Any amount other than what is needed by the body is released through the urine and symptoms of deficiency occur quickly if not taken in sufficient amounts and on a regular basis. Examples include the following vitamins:

B Vitamins are needed for the metabolism of proteins and fats as well as turning glucose into energy in the body and helping the skin, liver, hair, eyes and the nervous system. There are 8 B vitamins and they are:

B1 (thiamine) – helps with maintaining a healthy appetite and immune system. Needed for the production of energy in the body. Necessary to keep the cardiovascular and nervous systems functioning properly. Crucial part of the coenzyme that metabolizes carbohydrates.

Food Sources:
- nuts
- fish
- meats and other foods high in protein,
- wheat germ,
- peanut butter

Deficiencies appear as:
- Numbness and tingling in extremities
- Fatigue
- Depression
- Unable to focus and concentrate
- Problems with glucose metabolism
- Cramps in legs
- Paralysis in legs
- Problems with digestion

- Nausea
- Constipation
- Weight loss
- Appetite loss
- In severe cases, may cause heart failure

B2 (riboflavin) – helps to change folic acid and B6 in forms that are active in the body. Needed in production of energy as well as for growing, repairing and maintaining tissue.

Food Sources:
- milk
- cheese
- eggs
- liver
- green, leafy vegetables
- legumes
- nuts
- whole grains

Deficiencies appear as:
- Vision impairment
- Lips crack in the corners of mouth
- Dry, split and cracked lips
- Difficulty conceiving
- Diminished growth in children

B3 (niacin) – is known to help lower bad cholesterol and raise good cholesterol, increases circulation by dilating blood vessels. Helps digestive and nervous systems function properly as well as energy metabolism.

Food sources:
- eggs
- poultry
- nuts

- Vitamin enriched breads
- Avocados
- Legumes
- Collards
- Broccoli
- Bananas
- Seeds
- Tomatoes

Deficiencies appear as:
- Headaches
- Appetite loss
- Weight loss
- Irritability
- Depression
- Weakness
- Backache
- Tongue and mouth soreness
- Depression
- Fatigue
- Confusion

B5 (pantothenic acid) – necessary in producing red blood cells, helps the body with the use of riboflavin (B2) as well as the production of the steroid hormones. Regulates immune system

Food Sources:
- Sweet potatoes
- Meats
- Broccoli
- Kale
- Poultry
- Mushrooms
- eggs

Deficiencies appear as:

- Jittery nerves
- Skin problems
- Slowed metabolism

B6 (pyridoxine) -- helps form red blood cells, metabolizes amino and fatty acids and is necessary for the healthy function of the brain and its development. Helps metabolize glucose, fat and proteins, produces antibodies so is good for the immune system. Also important in the function of the nervous system.

<u>Food Sources:</u>
- nuts
- meats
- bananas
- avocado

<u>Deficiencies appear as:</u>
- kidney stones
- anemia
- confusion
- sore mouth
- depression
- confusion
- poor growth
- stomach pain

B7 (biotin) – helps to maintain normal blood sugar levels and contributes to managing metabolic responses. Well known for developing healthy hair, skin and nails.

<u>Food Sources:</u>
- milk
- nuts
- legumes
- mushroom
- salmon

- bananas
- carrots
- liver
- nutritional yeast
- chocolate (dark)

Deficiencies appear as:
- hair loss or thinning
- Pain in muscles
- Inflammation of skin
- Depression
- Alopecia
- Tingling in extremities

B9 folate (or folic acid –synthetic) – helps in the development of healthy brain function as well as one's mental health and stability. Works with B12 to in forming red blood cells and hemoglobin. It also contributes to the formation of DNA and RNA which is why is suggested that women increase their intake during pregnancy for the development of the baby.

Food Sources:
- green, leafy vegetables
- legumes
- beets
- oranges
- Cauliflower
- Broccoli
- Whole grains
- Brussel sprouts
- Carrots
- Okra
- Legumes

Deficiencies appears as:
- Pernicious anemia

- Fatigue
- Sore tongue

B12 (cobalamin) is needed to help break down amino and fatty acids, helps maintain health of nerve cells and create new cells. This vitamin is not available in plants. It can only be found in animal products. Methylcobalamin is the best source of cobalamin to use because it is a more natural form of B12, where cyanocobalamin is derived from a synthetic source.

Those who are strict vegetarians and vegans may need to supplement in order to receive a sufficient amount of B12. This vitamin is only absorbed in the intestine, however, it must be combined with a protein called the "intrinsic factor" found in gastric juices. The lack of this can lead to pernicious anemia.

Food Sources:
- milk
- eggs
- fish and
- meats
- Supplementation (injections, tablets or capsules or patches)
- It is sometimes added to cereals that have included additional vitamin/mineral sources

Deficiencies appear as:
- Pernicious anemia
- Problems walking
- Mental concerns
- Appetite loss
- Weight loss
- Tongue and mouth soreness

As you can see, many of the functions, foods and deficiencies of the B vitamins are the same. It is recommended to take a B-complex supplement to ensure you're getting a sufficient amount of all the

B's. Also, if you are taking a singular B vitamin over an extended period of time, this can affect the function of the other B's. Taking a B-complex ensures that you do not become deficient in or affect the other B's while taking a single B vitamin.

The other water soluble vitamin is:

Vitamin C (Ascorbic Acid) – this vitamin's benefits include assisting with the production of collagen which is necessary for healthy skin, ligaments and tendons, bones and the blood vessels. Contributes to wound healing. As an antioxidant, it is good for the immune system in the case of colds. It normalizes many of the most vital processes in the body.

Food Sources:
- oranges
- leafy green vegetables
- Brussel sprouts
- berries (blueberries, strawberries, raspberries)
- tomatoes
- cauliflower

Deficiencies appear as:
- anemia
- Joint pain
- Slow wound healing
- Problems with gums and teeth
- Problems with immune system

MINERALS – The body requires 2 types of minerals: macro-minerals and micro-minerals

Macro-minerals which are needed in the body in amounts of at least 100 mg/day. They are:

- *Calcium* – We're familiar with calcium's role in strengthening teeth and bones but it also plays a role in helping the blood clot, the transmission of nerves, as well as proper nerve and muscle function.
- *Phosphorus* – Is used in forming cells membranes and parts of the DNA. It also is used in making protein.
- *Iodine* -- Plays part in digestion, it is used in the production of hormones in the glands, helps to maintain proper blood pressure and volume.
- *Sodium* -- Plays many roles in the body such as regulation of blood pressure and aiding in the metabolizing of proteins and carbohydrates and helping with nerve transmission.
- *Potassium* – Helps keep blood pressure normal and aids in normal nerve transmission.
- *Sulfur* -- Helps in regulating blood sugar, relaxing nerves and muscles and producing collagen for joints and the skin.
- *Chloride* – Necessary for the proper balance of fluids and stomach acid
- *Magnesium* – Relaxes nerves and muscles, improves circulation and growth of bones. Helps metabolize some micro minerals and macro minerals.

Micro-minerals which are only needed in "trace" amounts but are necessary in order for the body to function properly. They are

- *Selenium* – Acts as an antioxidant
- *Iron* – Necessary in forming red blood cells and their function. Absorption of iron is increased with Vitamin C.
- *Chromium* – Regulates cholesterol, blood sugar and insulin.
- *Zinc* – Helps in many of the functions needed for development and growth including the making of DNA and cell growth, division and cell repair.
- *Boron* – Increases sex hormones in both men and women and metabolizing minerals that help form bones.
- *Manganese* – Is vital for the function and activity of several enzymes in the body.

- *Molybdenum* – Is also vital for the function and activity of several enzymes in the body.
- *Copper* – Helps with hemoglobin, collagen and elastin production.

This is a LOT of information to take in!!! Whoa! Now, the most important thing at this point is to concentrate on a few things at a time. Determine what you need and not try to go gung-ho and do too much at one time.

Your body plays a delicate balance between what it needs/requires and how to incorporate necessary changes into your lifestyle. Don't go out and buy a bunch of supplements and start taking them all at once. The body can only assimilate so much at a time. Not only can this make your feel worse but it can be a huge waste of time and money and in the end you may feel that making these positive changes in your life isn't worth it.

The first thing you want to do is to eat a balanced diet, then supplement as necessary. If you feel you are not getting a balance or a sufficient amount of nourishment, check with your doctor and/or health care professional if you are experiencing any problems with your health. Check to see if you have any imbalances or vitamin and mineral deficiencies. Should you decide to begin a vitamin/mineral regimen, start with the basics such as a high quality multi-vitamin/mineral. Take over a 1-3-month period to see if you notice any differences in your body, then if necessary, incorporate more.

When I look over the functions of many of these vitamins, especially the B vitamins, I can see why I experienced so many the problems. It appears I was severely malnourished in spite of the fact that I eat EVERYDAY, most of the time, 3 meals a day. However, I do recall I did not have a balanced diet, I eat plenty of sugary foods, too many carbohydrates, not nearly enough fruits and vegetables. No wonder I felt miserable so much and for so long on top of the other issues I experienced!!

BASIC NUTRIENTS

Carbohydrates - Cheapest, most efficient, and most readily available source of food energy in the world. There are 3 groups of carbohydrates:

- Monosaccharides (simple sugars)
  - Glucose
  - Fructose
  - Galactose
- Disaccharides
  - Sucrose
  - Lactose
  - maltose
- Complex carbohydrates
  - Starch
  - Dextrin
  - Glycogen
  - Fiber

Ways to improve use of carbohydrates in the body are:
- Eliminate or greatly reduce the use of processed foods
- Include more whole grains in the diet
- Eat more fresh fruits and vegetables
- Greatly reduce refined sugars and cereals
- Become a label reader – pay attention to any word that ends in "-ose", these are sugars (carbohydrates turn into sugar in the body)

Fats – made up of a combination of fatty acids and glycerol. There are 3 types of fats: saturated fatty acids, monosaturated fatty acids and polyunsaturated fatty acids.

- Saturated fatty acids
  - Generally, are solid at room temperature
  - Examples are chocolate, butter, cheese, coconut oil, palm oil
  - Whole milk
  - Cream
  - Can potentially increase cholesterol levels

- Monosaturated fatty acids

54

- o Do not become rancid very fast
- o Examples include peanuts, pecans, Brazil nuts, cashews, vegetable oil, olive oil
- o Reduce total cholesterol levels, mainly LDL (low density lipoprotein) (especially olive oil)

- Polyunsaturated fatty acids
  - o Generally, are liquid at room temperature
  - o Examples include corn, safflower, sunflower oils
  - o Walnuts
  - o Margarines
  - o Palm and coconut oils are exceptions because they are high in saturated fats
  - o Raises cholesterol and triglyceride levels

The benefits of fat include: 1) it provides energy to the body, 2) it is essential for every body cell, 3) helps body absorb certain vitamins (A, D, E, K), linoleic acid is supplied abundantly in dietary fat, and it increases palatability of foods (makes it taste good!).

Proteins -- Made up of building blocks called amino acids which consists of essential amino acids and non-essential amino acids.

Essential Amino Acids include:
- valine
- isoleucine
- leucine
- lysine
- methionine
- phenylalanine
- threonine
- tryptophan
- histidine (essential only for infants)

Since the body doesn't store amino acids, we need to supply a daily supply of these building blocks.

Non-Essential Amino Acids include:
- arginine
- glutamine
- tyrosine
- cysteine
- glycine
- proline
- serine
- ornithine
- alanine
- asparagine
- aspartate

The benefits of proteins include: 1) It is essential for growth, repair and maintenance of all body tissues, 2) takes part of enzymes and hormones to help regulate every important body function, 3) regulates water and acid base in body, 4) it is essential in formation of antibodies, so is critical in immune system function.

Even though I followed the traditional route of going to the doctor to have my symptoms addressed, no one addressed the cause of the symptoms. We live in such a "symptom-driven" health care system, that getting to the reason our bodies are responding to the imbalances is easily overlooked and neglected.

LINK #6

IN THE FIGHT FOR YOU:
YOUR IMMUNE SYSTEM

What exactly is immunity? According to Merriam-Webster Dictionary Online, immunity is *"the quality or state of being immune, especially a condition of being able to resist a particular disease especially through preventing development of a pathogenic microorganism or by counteracting the effects of its products"*.

When your emotions, mind and spirit are "out of whack" this lowers your immunity (resistance to illness, disease and STRESS). So it is extremely important that we keep our immune system up to par. Have you noticed when you are stressed you are more likely to catch a cold or the flu? If you are already dealing with dis-ease and/or illness, symptoms appear to become worse?

Our immune system is our first line of defense, like soldiers on the front line in war. It is there to ward off enemies and act as a warning that something is not quite right in the body. Reactions such as sneezing, coughing, infections, and even diarrhea, are some of the ways the body reacts to foreign matter.

Our bodies are created to naturally protect itself from foreign particles, substances and invaders. However, when flooded with impurities, whether from outside contaminants, stress or unhealthy emotions, the body's natural defense system can become overwhelmed and no longer recognizes foreign covered cells and begins to attack itself. There are hundreds of autoimmune diseases that stem from lowered immunity.

Have you noticed that when there's some type of virus, flu or cold going around in your office or your home that not everyone will get sick at the same degree as others? For example, Person #1 may become violently ill and it may take 2 weeks or more for them to fully recover. Person #2 will also get sick and take a week to recover. While Person #3 may only experience light symptoms and not become ill enough to stay home. Strictly speaking, if everyone is exposed to the germs equally, why doesn't everyone have the same symptoms for the same amount of time? Well, this is where the strength of each person's immune system comes into play.

Person #1 may already have a weakened immune system because they are already dealing with some auto-immune disorders such as diabetes, arthritis or are stressed out due personal issues. They also may not have the best eating habits, they drink a lot of caffeine and eat a lot of junk foods. All of these can make them more susceptible to viruses, colds, etc. because of a lowered immune system.

Person #2 may also be dealing with some health issues but tends to eat well and exercise sometimes but at the time this virus is going around is very stressed out and working a lot of overtime and is working to meet a deadline. Their immunity is lowered mainly due to stress. Again, this has made them more open to bacteria and viruses.

Person #3 has also been exposed to the virus but because they do not have any major health issues and tends to eat balanced meals, exercises, makes sure they get proper rest and manages the stressors in their life very well and has a positive attitude, their immune system is less vulnerable to foreign matters.

The above examples are just a few of the ways our immune systems can be compromised. There are many things to consider in keeping our bodies functioned as best it can.

My immune system was severely compromised over the years. I had more than one auto-immune deficiency disorder happening at the same time. I was given a diagnosis of multiple sclerosis but I actually was dealing with pernicious anemia (B^{12} deficiency), hypoglycemia AND amalgam (mercury) poisoning from the fillings in my teeth *(see chart in back of book)*. Even though I did not develop a lot of viruses and colds when I was at home, however, once I was around a lot of people for a long time, I would get colds, flus and viruses.

LYMPHATIC SYSTEM

The lymphatic system is a large part of the immune system and it is difficult to separate one from the other. What is the purpose of the lymphatic system? Why do you need to cleanse the lymphatic system?

In the case of "bad cells" invading the body, simply removing lymph nodes does not guarantee that dis-ease cannot, will not or has not spread to other organs (i.e., breast cancer, prostate cancer) because the toxins which have permeated in a particular organ or systems may have already spread to other organs or systems and may not manifest themselves for a very long time.

Lymph nodes are the filters that clean out the poisons and toxins in the body, but if they're clogged, they cannot move out of the body. Clogged lymph nodes are like trash sitting in the house in a corner for 20, 50, 60 or more years without ever emptying it. Can you imagine what your insides would look like? Yuck! To clarify effects of a toxic lymphatic system, think of the following conditions:

- Swelling/fluid retention (feet, knees, ankles, legs)
- Infections
- Sore throat/laryngitis
- Leukemia
- Cancer
- Tonsillitis
- Chronic fatigue
- Pleurisy
- Colds/flu/pneumonia
- Emphysema
- PMS
- Mononucleosis (glandular fever)
- Lymphoma

These are manifestations of lymphatic congestion and buildup of poisons as well as lack of a healthy diet. Do you or anyone you know suffer or ever suffered from any of the above complaints or dis-eases? By the time symptoms appear, toxins may have been building up in the body for weeks, months and even YEARS!

Externally, the skin serves as part of the immune system by protecting us from pollutants in the air that we are exposed to on a daily basis.

The immune system works "behind the scenes" by acting as soldiers on the front line of defense to keep your body and cells protected from enemies such as germs, bacteria and other poisons that enter the system as well as driving off dead cell die-off internally and externally. Keep your soldiers STRONG!!

LINK #7

IT ALL BALANCES OUT:
ACID/ALKALINE BALANCE

What IS acid and alkaline? Acidity and alkalinity are determined on a 14-point (pH) scale (p = power, H = hydrogen) with "0" being most acidic and 14 being most alkaline. Seven (7) is considered neutral. Different organs and body systems require different levels of acid and alkaline. These measurements generally balance each other out.

How does the body maintain acid/alkaline balance? Mainly through the food choices we make. Foods are either acid, alkaline or a balance of the two. Our blood has about a stable pH of 7.41.

When we eat foods that are too acidic, it affects our blood and kidneys through the colon, kidneys and other body parts, systems and eliminative organs (skin, mucous membranes, sinuses). Therefore, the more alkaline foods we eat such as fruits and vegetables, the better off we are. Below is a list of foods based on acid, alkaline and balance according to Elson Haas in his book entitled, "Staying Healthy with Nutrition".

Alkaline Foods
- All vegetables
- Majority of fruits
- Millet
- Buckwheat
- Sprouted Beans
- Sprouted Seeds
- Olive Oil
- Soaked Almonds

Balanced
- Brown Rice

- Corn
- Soybeans
- Lima Beans
- Almonds
- Sunflower Seeds
- Brazil Nuts
- Honey
- Most dried beans and peas
- Tofu
- Nonfat Milk
- Vegetable Oils

Acid
- Wheat
- Oats
- White Rice
- Pomegranates
- Strawberries
- Cranberries
- Breads
- Refined Flour
- Refined Sugar
- Cashews, pecans and peanuts
- Milk
- Cheeses
- Eggs
- Fish
- Poultry

Based on the Standard American Diet (SAD) – ISN'T IT?!! – most of us are overly acidic. Let's look for the middle ground in this and understand that we must do the best we can to keep our bodies in a position to heal and ward off dis-ease.

Keeping the pH balance in the body can affect the health in areas such as energy levels, digestion, heart health, hormonal balance, ability to gain or loss weight, immunity, bones, bowel health, and urinary function.

The best ways to measure the body's acid/alkaline levels are through the urine and saliva. To get an idea to find your body's pH level is to test it first thing in the morning – before eating any food or brushing your teeth. Then measure again about 3 hours after a meal. Try testing about twice a week to get a better take on what your normal pH levels are.

Testing the urine pH can show whether the body is utilizing minerals such as potassium, sodium, calcium and magnesium. These minerals help the body balance and keep acid levels in check. If the body produces too much acid or alkaline, it will attempt to get rid of any excess through the urine. The pH level of urine should be somewhere between 6.0 and 7.0.

Saliva pH levels should fluctuate between 6.5 to 6.8, anything below this indicates the body is overproducing acids.

How do you test your pH levels?
Through the use of pH strips which can be dipped in urine and/or swabbed on the tongue. By looking at the resulting color, you can see your pH level. There should be a diagram of the pH levels from acidic to alkaline on the bottle of strips or you can purchase a chart that has the color range of the pH levels. Your pH changes throughout the day depending on what you eat or drink. Test your urine and/or saliva in the morning and evening for a couple days a week to determine your average pH level.

Ways to Keep pH Levels in Balance:
- Eat more foods with fiber
- Dry Skin Brushing (see chapter
- Drink sufficient amount of water daily
- Eat a sufficient amount of fruits and vegetables
- Get the correct amount of vitamins and minerals

LINK #8

LET'S GET TOGETHER: FOOD COMBINATION SYSTEM

Food combining is a concept that says in order to obtain the best possible digestion and use of the foods we eat, there are particular "rules" that must be observed and followed. These rules say that certain foods should be eaten together, alone or in combination with others. While other combinations may cause acid reflux, indigestion, constipation, diarrhea and other digestive issues.
Here's a brief and simplified layout of food combining.

- Fruits should be eaten alone (wait at least 20 minutes to 1 hour before eating other foods).

- Watermelon and melons should be eaten separate from other fruits.

- Vegetables should be eaten with protein OR starch, but proteins and starches should not be eaten together – Oops! There goes that hamburger on a bun! DO NOT EAT STARCH and PROTEINS IN THE SAME MEAL!

- During the digestion process, certain enzymes are utilized to break down different foods. Fruits take little digestion time because they are alkaline and break down quickly in the stomach. However, when combined with other foods that may be acid, it causes the fruit to stay in the stomach longer where it ferments and causes gas as it passes through the intestines.

When proteins, which are acid, and starches, which are alkaline are combined they interfere with how the other is utilized and this slows down digestion. This also causes digestion problems such as gas, acid reflux, poor digestion, and underutilization of nutrients.

Following a food combining regimen *does* require that you eat "consciously" and make healthy choices. Even if you don't follow these rules 100% of the time, begin to incorporate them into your lifestyle. Results can be obtained such as less gas and stomach upset, better assimilation of foods and possibly weight loss.

In order to make the most of this system, you should:

- Take food enzymes
- Avoid process foods
- Avoid white potatoes, rice and other starchy foods
- Eat more fruits and vegetables, but eat very moderately from starchy vegetables (potatoes, peas, carrots, potatoes)
- Eat whole grains (breads, cereals)

LINK #9

SPICING IT UP WITH HERBS: COMMON KITCHEN HERBS AND SPICES FOR YOUR HEALTH

What are herbs? They are simply highly nutritious foods that contain high sources of various vitamins and minerals. Herbs have been around since the beginning of time. The Bible even mentions herbs 133 times!

There are many herbs that are used as seasonings in our daily cooking. However, the nutritional value of these herbs and spices are often overlooked. I teach a class based on the title of this chapter "Spicing It Up with Herbs". In this class, participants have the opportunity to taste each herb or spice separately to bring an awareness of the effect it has on the senses – the taste, feel, look, and sometimes its immediate physical effect on the body.

Now while in the kitchen cooking and seasoning your favorite foods, know that you are not just seasoning for taste but also for the benefits you may receive from using herbs. If you're looking at cutting down on sodium, most herbs have a natural sodium content that does not have a negative effect on blood pressure. So your foods do not have to be bland and tasteless to be delicious and healthy!

Below are a few of the most common herbs found in your spice rack, along with the origins of the herb, its potential physical effect, vitamin/mineral content and some foods or dishes it may add to. *(Refer to Appendix for explanation of the properties of each herb.)*

<u>Basil</u> – This herb finds its origins in India with a distinctive odor and sharp taste. The properties of basil are as an antispasmodic, antibacterial, antidepressant, adrenal stimulant as well as soothing digestion. Potential effects include relief of nervous tension, including tension headaches, stress, and indigestion.

The parts of the herb that are considered medicinal are fresh and/or dried. Basil is very high in Vitamins A & K. Foods that use basil include tomatoes, garlic, olives, salads, stews are vegetables, pasta, meat, and poultry.

Cayenne (Capsicum) Fruit – Originated in South America, cayenne has a pungent, bitter and acrid taste. Its medicinal properties are as a stimulant, tonic, carminative, diaphoretic, rubefacient, antiseptic, anti-bacterial, thermogenic.

Cayenne may stimulate blood circulation, purify blood, promote fluid elimination and sweat, as well act as a nerve stimulant. Vitamin and mineral content includes vitamin C, folic acid, niacin and zinc. Can be used in Mexican and Cajun dishes or In most foods depending on taste.

Chives: It is believed to have originated in Central Asia. Related to the onion family but flavor is less dominant and subtle. It acts as an anti-neoplastic, antioxidant, antibiotic and can be used as a digestive and appetite stimulant.

The medicinal parts of chives come from the grass and seeds. The vitamin content includes vitamins A and C, potassium, calcium, and folic acid. Some foods chives are used in include salads, potatoes, and eggs.

Cinnamon – Ancient Egyptians and Chinese used this herb thousands of years ago. It acts as a carminative, diaphoretic, astringent, stimulant, antimicrobial, antifungal, antibacterial. Cinnamon may promote digestion, relieve nausea, vomiting, diarrhea, upset stomach and Irritable Bowel Syndrome (IBS). It may also help the body utilize insulin more efficiently. The medicinal part is the bark. Cinnamon is used in pies, oatmeal, tea, toast, apple cider.

Clove – Indigenous to Philippines and Molucca Islands, it has a hot, slightly sweet taste. Its actions include acting as an antioxidant, anesthetic, anti-inflammatory, anodyne, antispasmodic, carminative, stimulant, prevents vomiting, antihistamine, as well as a thermogenic.

It may help with asthma, bronchitis, nausea, vomiting, flatulence, diarrhea, hypothermia, and an antiparasitic. The seeds and/or flower buds contain its medicinal components. Cloves are used in cider, apples, and lamb.

Cumin – Used in ancient Greece and Rome, it has a slightly bitter pepper taste with a hint of citrus. Cumin acts as a stimulant, soothing digestion, antispasmodic, diuretic, and may increase milk in breastfeeding. It also may help with indigestion and flatulence.

The seeds contain its medicinal properties. It is high in protein, potassium, iron and thiamine. Dishes such as lamb, chicken, beef, Mexican, Indian and Middle Eastern.

Fennel – Used by Greeks and has a fragrant odor and warm, subtle, sweet licorice-like taste. Its actions are as an antacid, soothing diuretic, anti-inflammatory, anti-spasmodic, soothing digestive, mild expectorant, an appetite suppressant.

Helps support healthy digestion, relieves occasional gas and menstrual discomfort. Fennel may help with indigestion, flatulence, increase of milk flow in breastfeeding, relief of colic in babies when taken by nursing mothers.

The whole plant and seeds of fennel contains its medicinal properties. It is high in magnesium and vitamin A, iron, calcium, selenium and phosphorus. Fennel is used on fish, Italian dishes, lamb chops and meatloaf.

Fenugreek – Beneficial in helping with digestion and maintaining the lymphatic system.

Garlic – Goes all the way back to ancient Chinese traditions. Its strong, pungent odor and taste has anti-microbial, antibiotic, cardio-protective, hypotensive, anti-carcinogen, promotes sweating, reduces blood pressure, anti-coagulant, lowers blood cholesterol levels, lowers blood sugar levels, expectorant, digestive stimulant, diuretic, anti-histamine, antispasmodic.

Garlic may inhibit cancer cell formation and proliferation, lower serum total and low density lipoprotein cholesterol; may also help stimulate immune system; protect organs from damage induced by synthetic drugs, chemical pollutants and the effects of radiation. The bulb contains the medicinal component. The root contains potassium and vitamin C. Garlic is used in sauces, spaghetti, and actually can be used in most foods.

Ginger – Its actions include anti-nausea, relieves headaches and arthritis, anti-inflammatory, circulatory stimulant, expectorant, antispasmodic, antiseptic, diaphoretic, guards against blood clots, peripheral vasodilator, prevents vomiting, carminative, antioxidant.

Ginger may stimulate blood flow to the digestive system, calm nausea and morning sickness, prevent vomiting, increase the absorption of nutrients, increase action of the gallbladder, while protecting the liver against toxins and prevent the formation of ulcers. May be used for flatulence, circulation problems, impotence, and prevention of nausea after chemotherapy.

The medicinal part of ginger is the root. Its vitamin and mineral components are calcium, magnesium, manganese, potassium, phosphorus and vitamin C. Some of the foods garlic is used with include chicken, lamb, vegetables, breads, baked goods, fish, and fruits.

Parsley – Acts as an antioxidant, tonic, digestive, and diuretic. It may help expel excess water (by flushing the kidneys). It is one of the richest food sources of vitamin C. Parsley also contains calcium, copper, iron, potassium, and vitamin A.

The leaves contain its medicinal properties and is used in dishes such as potatoes, fish, pasta and chicken.

Rosemary – Some of its actions include being an antioxidant, anti-inflammatory, astringent, nervine, carminative, antiseptic, diuretic, diaphoretic, promotion of bile flow, anti-depressant, circulatory stimulant, anti-spasmodic, nervous system and cardiac tonic.

It may act as an effective food preservative, may also be effective in preventing breast cancer, fights against deterioration of brain functions (improves memory), is useful in treatment of migraine and tension headaches, nervous tension, flatulence, depression, chronic fatigue syndrome and joint pain.

The whole plant has medicinal properties. The vitamin and mineral content includes calcium, iron, potassium, phosphorus, magnesium, zinc, manganese, Vitamin A and C, folic acid. Rosemary is used in foods such as potatoes, stuffing, chicken, Italian dishes, lamb, and vegetables.

Sage – Its actions include antioxidant, antimicrobial, antibiotic, antiseptic, carminative, and antispasmodic. It may help kill bacteria and fungi; may be used as a gargle for sore throat, laryngitis and mouth ulcers, helps reduce breast milk production, relieve night sweats and hot flashes of menopause.

The leaf is the part that contains medicinal properties. The vitamin and mineral components include magnesium, calcium, potassium, high in zinc, sodium, thiamine, Vitamin A and C. Sage is used in dressing, chicken, sausage and green beans.

Thyme – Its actions include that of an antioxidant, expectorant, antiseptic, antispasmodic, astringent, tonic, antimicrobial, antibiotic, wound healer, carminative, calms coughs, and nervine. It may help with deep seated chest infections such as chronic coughs and bronchitis, sinusitis, laryngitis, asthma and irritable bowel syndrome.

Its leaves, which contain chromium, iron, magnesium, silicon, sodium, Vitamin A, and zinc. Foods it's used in include chicken, dressing, sausage, fish, beef, and Italian dishes.

Turmeric – Its actions include that as an antioxidant, anti-inflammatory antimicrobial, antibacterial, antifungal, antiviral, anticoagulant, and analgesic.

Turmeric may also reduce cholesterol, reduce post-exercise pain, heal wounds, antispasmodic, protect liver cells, increase bile production and flow. It may inhibit colon and breast cancer, nausea, digestive disturbances, and where the gall bladder has been removed, use in hepatitis, boosts insulin activity, reduce the risk of stroke, help in rheumatoid arthritis, cancer, candida, AIDS, Chrohn's disease, eczema, and digestive problems.

The whole herb is used medicinally. Chicken, lamb, Middle Eastern dishes, curry dishes, rice are some of the dishes that include turmeric in recipes.

Here is a list of some additional herbal dietary supplements that are not commonly known or used in our kitchen cabinets but are also beneficial in keeping the body in balance due to their vitamin and mineral content. Most herbal supplements have various desired effects on different body systems. These are by no means a list of ALL the many herbal foods that are at our disposal.

Alfalfa – It's origins are in the Middle East. It is considered the "Father of all foods" by Arabs. Has the highest amount of chlorophyll of any plant known to man. This is important because chlorophyll's composition is nearly the same as humans.   content its leaves contain a high beta-carotene content and has 8 of the essential amino acids which are needed for protein production. Alfalfa also contains, magnesium, potassium and calcium and vitamins, A, C, D, E and K.

The plant's vitamin C content is 4 times higher than that of an orange. It also is rich in calcium, B12 (which can be of huge benefit to vegans and vegetarians who may have difficulty getting a sufficient amount in their diets).   Studies have shown Alfalfa may be beneficial for diabetes, high cholesterol, joint comfort, and upset stomach.

Astragalus – Is a Chinese medicine herb. Some studies indicate it may support T-Cell function, may be a protector of the liver from damage caused by chemotherapy in cancer patients. May greatly benefit the immune system, adrenals and digestion.

Although it can be considered an immune system builder, it should not be used for all illnesses. Individuals suffering from known infections and other autoimmune issues should not use this herb because it may increase the activity of the virus.

Bayberry – Benefits the health of the sinuses, respiratory system as well as the female reproductive system. Its best quality is its calming and soothing effect on mucous membranes especially in the digestive and respiratory tracts. It may be beneficial to the female system by helping to check menstrual imbalances.

Bee Pollen – Beneficial for immunity, energy and adrenals support, specifically used for reduction of allergies and respiratory concerns. It contains a nearly perfect balance of vitamins, minerals, essential amino acids, carbohydrates, fats, proteins and the necessary enzyme precursors.

Black Cohosh – Beneficial in relief of menstrual discomfort, helps calm nervous system, hormonal balancer for men and women. For women it may help reduce or eliminate hot flashes, mood swings and those suffering from night sweats. Isn't that a relief for those going through the marvelous change of life called menopause!

Mothers-to-be must be cautious not to take during pregnancy due to its ability to cause contraction of the uterus. May be used in late stage or near term to help with labor, but only under the direction of a qualified health care professional.

Most people think of Black Cohosh mainly for women and female issues, however, it may also have an effect on the respiratory system by loosening up mucous.

Use of Black Cohosh should be limited to no more than 6 months because it may cause issues such as joint pain, vomiting, blood pressure problems (low) or dizziness. Only under the direction of a health care professional should it be taken beyond 6 months.

Black Walnut – Provides oxygen to the cells.   This action can contribute to the killing of parasites and expulsion of pinworms, tapeworms and ringworms from the intestinal system.   It can also help rid the body of candida.   It has a laxative effect on the system.

Burdock -- Helps support liver, kidneys, skin and lymphatic systems. It is an excellent blood cleanser and purifier. Burdock contains a substance called inulin which is beneficial in the metabolizing carbohydrates. Great for dispelling poisons from the body through the lymphatic system.

Cascara Sagrada – Beneficial for occasional constipation and is not considered to be habit forming. It can improve the peristaltic action of the intestines due to its calming effect on the autonomic nervous system. It may also increase bile action in the liver and gallbladder which Is needed for proper elimination.

Chaste Tree Berry – Beneficial in the relief of hot flashes and menopause discomfort

Chickweed – Beneficial as a general tonic for good health including weight loss, joint support and comfort and inflammation. Helps dissolve fatty substances from the body both internally and externally including cellulite.

Crampbark – Helps alleviate cramping anywhere in the body but it is known especially for reducing cramping in the uterus and stomach. This makes it great to use during menstruation.   It can have a calming effect on the uterus and ovaries making it beneficial pain during menstruation.

Damiana – Beneficial in increasing sexual desire. Although mainly known to help balance hormones in women, it is also effective for men also. Other uses include having a laxative effect on children as well as a cough suppressant.

Dandelion – Beneficial for maintenance of healthy skin, eyes, liver, kidneys and blood. Beneficial for digestive support as well as for liver and gallbladder health. It also acts a natural diuretic.

Echinacea – Beneficial for strengthening the immune system. Known to help shorten the during of a cold. But should only be used for a limited amount of time. When use over an extended period of time, its effectiveness is diminished.

Flax – Helps maintain healthy cholesterol levels that are already in the normal range, also helps with occasional constipation as well as strengthening the entire body for overall good health.

Gota Kola –Beneficial in helping to improve memory. Also benefits maintenance of a healthy.

Kelp – Helps in thyroid function and maintenance as well as overall health.

Licorice – Its use has been known since ancient times in both New and Old Worlds. Licorice has a sweet taste/flavor. Its actions are as a gentle laxative, tonic, anti-inflammatory, anti-bacterial, anti-arthritic. It is known to soothe gastric and intestinal mucous membranes, and an expectorant.

Licorice may provide nutrients to almost all body systems; detoxify, is a natural sweetener, regulate blood sugar levels and recharge depleted adrenal glands, help heal peptic ulcers, soothe irritated membranes and loosen and expel phlegm in the upper respiratory tract, treat sore throat, assist with urinary tract infections, coughs, bronchitis, gastritis and constipation.

The root contains its medicinal properties and is high in chromium, iron, magnesium, vitamin C and zinc. Licorice is used as a tea or dried root sticks.

Marshmallow -- Helps to maintain healthy mucus membranes. Helps sooth irritated and inflamed internal membranes such as the gastro-intestinal tract, lungs, colon, bladder/urinary tract.

Milk Thistle – Supports function and maintenance of liver and gallbladder.

Passion Flower – Helps to relieve occasional muscle spasms as well as discomfort related to menopause. It acts as a nervine and is calming, helps relax muscles and nerves.

Red Raspberry – Beneficial for relief of occasional stomach discomfort as well as overall female health. This herb is acts a balancer throughout a woman's life – from puberty, pregnancy, pre- and post-menopause. Has been used for children in case of colds

Reishi Mushroom – Benefits the immune system and supports blood pressure already within normal range.

Royal Jelly – Beneficial for glandular including adrenal support as well as menopausal discomfort.

Sarsaparilla –Beneficial in providing nourishment to maintain healthy skin and good health.

Saw Palmetto – Helps to maintain a healthy prostate.

Valerian – Helps support healthy cardiovascular and nervous systems.

Wild Cherry Bark -- Beneficial for a healthy respiratory system.

Yellow Dock – Beneficial tonic for skin and lymphatic systems.

LINK #10

THE ELIXIR OF LIFE!:
IMPORTANCE OF WATER

Just how does water work in the body? Every function in the body is regulated and monitored by having an efficient amount of water. All of our cells contain and are surrounded by water. There must be enough water in the body in order to be able to transport the necessary elements, chemicals, hormones and nutrients to our vital organs for them to function effectively and efficiently.

Many times when we think we are hungry, we are actually THIRSTY!! Our bodies are composed of approximately 75% water, only about 25% of our body is solid mass! By the time your body signals that you're thirsty, you are already dehydrated!

Some areas of the body, for example, the brain is composed of 85% water. The brain is most vulnerable to becoming dehydrated and easily depleted of water. If you're having foggy thinking or unable to concentrate, try drinking water.

When there is a lack of water, the body begins to "cry" out with symptoms such as pain, discomfort, and ultimately with "dis-ease". Just as we are well aware our body needs certain nutrients, vitamins and minerals in order to ward off illness and to keep the body functioning at its optimal capacity, water should be added high on this list as well. In fact, in order to guarantee that the body can absorb nutrients, vitamins, minerals, etc., there must be adequate water available.

Another important part of the body that is in high need of hydration is the lower back which tends to suffer from pain and discomfort. Seventy-five percent (75%) of the upper body's weight is supported by the water volume in the 5th spinal lumbar disc. I've heard of many cases of people suffering for years with lower back pain without any lasting results.

Many people end up having surgery to resolve the issues when it is possible that just consuming more water may have been of some benefit. So the next time you feel minor pain or twitch in your body, maybe drinking more water first can bring some relief. (NOTE: Always consult your health care professional for any diagnosis or treatments).

How do you know if you're drinking enough water on a daily basis? Ideally, drink half the body's weight in ounces of water every day, i.e., a 160 lb. person would drink 80 ounces. If consuming caffeine products (soda, coffee, chocolate) add an additional 2 ounces of water to each ounce of caffeine consumed. For example, for every 8 ounces of coffee, drink an extra 16 ounces of water).

When speaking of drinking water, I'm talking about JUST water, not juice, tea, coffee or any other liquid. Even though these drinks contain water, they are NOT WATER!!! Whenever you add another food or substance to water – it is no longer water – it is FOOD! The body then goes into the digestive process by breaking down and separating the substance from the water in the stomach, colon and kidneys. This requires more water and activity which further adds to the dehydration of the body.

There is so much controversy or mindsets of which water is the best to consume. Should you drink distilled, reverse osmosis, spring, alkaline, deionized water or just tap water? There are reasons pro and con for drinking or not drinking each of these. This could take up another book to sort all of this out. Instead I will focus on WHY you should drink water.

Reasons to Drink Water and Keep the Body Hydrated:
- Drinking water first thing in the morning to replace water absorbed overnight
- Drink water approximately 30 minutes prior to eating a meal. This helps prepare the digestive tract for the process of assimilating food and helps those who may be having digestive issues such as colitis, indigestion, heartburn and other concerns.

- Drinking water 2 to 2.5 hours after a meal to continue the digestion process and replaces the water used to help break food down.
- Those who have don't consume sufficient vegetables and fruits and have problems with constipation should drink 2 to 3 glasses first thing in the morning. This can act as a natural laxative due to is lubricating effects on the colon and provides the moisture needed to allow for a "smooth move"!
- Whenever you feel thirsty, preferably before then, you should drink water.

If you are not drinking enough water, don't try to go from zero to 100 immediately! Gradually increase your water intake over time. Also do not try to drink your daily suggested amount of water all at once. You would not consume all your meals at once because the stomach would become overwhelmed and you wouldn't feel very well! This is the same with water consumption, spread your intake throughout the day. By spreading it out you allow the body to absorb and utilize the water better.

MAKE WATER YOUR MEDICINE!!

Take it as if your life depends on it – because it may!!

LINK #11

JUST A FEW BRUSH STROKES AWAY!:
DRY SKIN BRUSHING

We're moving right along and now a way to *"exercise"* the internal body with a few brush strokes!

The skin is the *LARGEST EXTERNAL* and one of the most important eliminative organs in the body. The Skin is also known as the "3rd kidneys" (the lungs are known as the "2nd kidneys"). Nearly 25% of all toxins released from the body come through the skin surface. Isn't it great to know that we are blessed to have more than the one set of kidneys?!

Dry Skin Brushing is a simple process that increases circulation on top of the skin and allows improved release of toxins by allowing pores to remain open. The outcome is increased ability to fight off bad bacteria, and at the same time the skin appears and feels firmer while helping your skin look and feel healthier and more elastic!

Possible benefits of Dry Skin Brushing include:

- Getting rid of layers of dead surface skin
- Firming and tightening of skin
- Diminishing or eliminating cellulite
- Detoxifying of Lymphatic System
- Improving digestion.
- Immune system is stronger and more resistant to dis-ease and bacteria
- Fueling Circulation
- _ALL Body Systems_ operating at much higher level

Wow! Now does all that beat the cost of those risky, expensive surgeries, tummy tucks, liposuction that do not provide a permanent solution to the problem? Dry skin brushing is not a miracle method either, it must be done consistently and over time to obtain its long-term benefits. Aren't you worth the Time?! We're talking about 5-10 minutes out of your day – every day!

HOW TO USE A DRY SKIN BRUSH?

- Always use an ALL NATURAL, 100% VEGETABLE brush (synthetic brushes tend to scratch or bruise the skin surface) with a long, removable handle to help reach parts of the body that are not easy to reach – the back, for example.

- Dry skin brush, BEFORE Showering or Bathing, at least ONCE per day. Twice is ideal.

- If you are going to exercise in the morning, dry skin brush BEFORE working out, otherwise the skin will be wet or damp from sweating and you don't want to use the brush on wet or damp skin. When the skin is wet, brushing will stretch the skin, which is the opposite of what you want to happen.

- Remember to brush towards the Heart.

- Using LONG strokes, brush each part of the body several times 2-3 times BRISKLY and COMPLETELY. Start lightly until you adjust to use of brush. Brush the WHOLE Body being careful not to irritate the skin.

- *Don't use on broken, bruised or damaged skin.*

- Begin by brushing the soles of the Feet in a circular motion. Every body part and system is represented in the feet (reflexology areas),

- Then go to calves, and outer and inner thighs using long, smooth strokes.

- Next, using circular motion, brush stomach beginning on the lower right side (the liver and ascending colon area), up and across the solar plexus region (the transcending colon and the top of the liver) and down the left side (the descending colon) as well as the middle of the stomach and buttocks.

- Do LIGHT Strokes over and around breast. Women, DO NOT brush the nipples (they tend to be very sensitive).

- Lightly brush neck on both sides (including under chin -- lymph glands are here), then across both shoulders.

- Finally brush palms and back of hands up to the arms including underarms (more lymphatic glands here!).

- Take a WARM Bath or Shower, with a "chaser" of a COOL water by rinsing at the end to stimulate blood circulation and keep surface of skin warm. It may take a little time to adjust to doing this but it is so refreshing afterwards!

- To keep brush clean, wash brush every few weeks in water and let it dry completely before using again.

This may seem like a lot to do in 5-10 minutes and may take longer initially until you get the hang of it. Once you get into the habit, it's like brushing your teeth! ☺

LINK #12

LET'S GET MOVING!:
THE POWER OF REBOUNDING

Exercise is about movement. Movement that can extend the life span by revving the body up to burn fat, increase energy, rid the body of toxins (through the lymphatic system, skin, bowels, bladder), increase heart rate, stimulate the cardiovascular system - to name a few of many benefits.

There are different types of exercise and even more benefits! Usually when it comes to exercise, think of fitness clubs, running, walking, biking, aerobics, yoga, Pilates and other forms of exercise. Exercise also includes flexibility, strength, endurance as well as speed.

You may not want or are able to be a marathon runner, however, there is SOME type of movement you can do according to your physical ability and capability to improve the state of your health and physical well-being.

I recommend that you consult a fitness professional (as well as your doctor) to determine and put together a fitness program to suit your individual needs.

There are many wonderful forms and types of exercise that we can do to get our bodies in great shape such as running, walking, cycling, aerobics, Zumba, free weights – all are excellent forms of exercise and are recommended depending upon what you're looking to achieve.

However, there's another great form of exercise known as rebounding on a mini-trampoline (also called rebounder). No special clothing is required such as gym shoes, sweat pants – just light and comfortable apparel – no shoes required! (Right up my alley – love being barefoot! Rebounding can be done while watching TV or listening to your favorite music.

This simple form of exercise and its extensive benefits are often overlooked because it seems TOO simple! It is not only beneficial to flush out old waste products from the body, but also a way to exercise without putting a strain on the knees (compared to running or walking on a hard surface).

Rebounding can positively affect every joint and cell in the body. Most importantly, it is FUN!

Some of the Major Benefits of Rebounding include:
• Strengthens entire body
• Aids lymphatic circulation
• Stimulates metabolism
• Increases the capacity of breathing
• Circulates more oxygen to the tissues
• Helps prevent cardiovascular disease
• Enhances digestion and eliminative processes
• Helps normalize blood pressure
• Takes stress off joints and bones
• Helps increase production of red blood cells
• Lowers elevated cholesterol and triglyceride levels
• Tones glandular system – especially thyroid
• Improves overall body coordination
• Increases muscle tone
• Improves digestion and elimination
• Relieves menstrual comfort
• Tends to slow down the aging process
• Boosts immunity
• Reduces body fat
• Almost everyone can benefit from it

How to Use Rebounder
• Stand in middle of trampoline – without shoes – make sure you maintain good balance

- Without lifting feet, gently bounce for about 5 minutes to activate lymphatic fluid flow (help body release toxins)
- If someone is disabled or unable to stand, place their feet on rebounder while someone else bounces, both will gain benefits from this. Get those little ones bouncing for you, they'll love it!
- The rebounder can be used as cardiac exercise by walking or running in place for 20-30 minutes.

If you have never used a rebounder before I suggest you start with the gentle "health bounce". This is done by placing the feet firmly and not lifting them from the mat while the body "bounces" up and down. This health bounce is sufficient to obtain all the benefits of rebounding while gently strengthening the entire body.

Adults can start with 5 minutes of rebounding and increase their time as their fitness level improves. Seniors can start with 2 minutes several times per day, with at least 30 minutes between rebounding sessions.

It's necessary for older people to start gradually in order to give the connective tissue holding the internal organs in place time to strengthen. This prevents the possibility of "prolapsed organs" – the only possible negative effect to rebounding reported in the medical literature. Therefore, increase your rebounding time gradually.

Because rebounding is an exercise that can reduce body fat – and gives your body energy when it's tired, jump on your rebounder when you NEED energy, not just when you HAVE energy!

LINK #13

CAN YOU FEEL IT!!
ENERGY – SELF-HEALING
TECHNIQUES

What is ENERGY?! According to Merriam-Webster online, energy is expressed in the following ways:

- dynamic quality (narrative energy); the capacity of acting or being active (intellectual energy); a usually positive spiritual force (the energy flowing through all people)

- vigorous exertion of power; vigor (investing time and energy)

- a fundamental entity of nature that is transferred between parts of a system in the production of physical change within the system and usually regarded as the capacity for doing work

- usual power (as heat or electricity); also, the resources for producing such power

In addition to healing the body through the use of herbs, vitamins, water and nutrition, ENERGY also has a tremendous effect on our health. The way energy flows through or is blocked in the body can result in a positive or negative response in one's wellbeing. This can include understanding how our body responds to stress, reducing pain, how we assimilate food – including the foods we eat through our bodies, thoughts, emotions, spirit as well as the electromagnetic fields we are exposed to daily.

Here are some ways energy exists in our lives:

Wiping/Cutting Off Negative Energy
Sometimes we come into contact with people with negative attitudes, even our own negative attitudes, thoughts can cause us to

become stressed and upset. To quickly get rid of this negativity, start from your head down to your feet by making a sweeping, fanning motion down to your feet, making a sweeping motion down the front of your body. Do this 2-3 times. DO NOT sweep upward – only from top – down.

Stretching

Get in the habit of stretching at least 10-15 minutes a day. When we wake up in the morning our bodies may be stiff. By gently stretching the neck, arms, legs and other body parts, we relax the muscles and release energy that helps us through the day and clears the brain for better thinking and mood.

Breathing

Most people shallow breath – that is only breathing from the chest up. By learning to breathe from the stomach up through the diaphragm we reduce tension, pain, stress and more. Learning to breath correctly opens up oxygen in our cells which provides more energy to the body.

Calories

Used to measure not only the energy used by the body, but also to tell us the amount of energy present in food. When eating the healthy, live foods, the nutrition gained increases our energy levels.

Basal Metabolic Rate (BMR)

This is energy used even when lying down completely relaxed, awake, or even on an empty stomach and is essential just to maintain life. It is measured by multiplying bodyweight in pounds' times 10 (ex. 160 lbs. x 10 = 1600 calories/day.

Energy from Electromagnetic Fields

Today we are surrounded by, relying on and depending on so many electronic products to function day to day in the air, from telephone wires, cell towers, computers, cell phones, microwave ovens, medical testing devices and more.

Twenty to 30 years ago, there were only a few electric devices in our homes. We had televisions, stereos, radios, in our kitchens we had blenders, toasters, stoves, refrigerators, microwave ovens and maybe a few other items.

However, today, we have many devices that we use to function and accomplish many tasks. Everyone has their own cell phones, most of us use computers, Ipads, smartphones, Bluetooth, gaming devices, digital televisions, cable boxes and remote controls in every room of the house.

All of these devices emit energy through electromagnetic fields that affect our bodies, which by the way, also consists of electromagnetic fields! Our body parts and systems operate on different frequencies in order for them to function properly such as the heart and the brain.

Frequent exposure to so much electromagnetic energy can disrupt the natural flow of energy in the body and create dis-ease and dysfunction. One way to protect yourself from the negative energy that surrounds us is to use a device called a "diode" which directs currents AWAY from the body so that it does not absorb the negative energy. They come in the form a necklace or a device that you place on or near your body.

Testing fruits and vegetables for good energy
Just as our bodies have energy, all living things have energy, including the foods we eat. When buying fresh fruits and vegetables, hold your hand lightly over the food item, when you feel a sensation of warmth, it has good energy. This is the one you want to choose. This feeling may not happen when the produce is GMO (genetically modified).

Use these suggestions on a daily basis combined with other healthy choices and you will begin to see your outlook on life improve gradually but significantly!

There are many simple, easy-to-use techniques that can be applied at almost anytime and anywhere. These techniques only take a few minutes of your time and can gradually assist the body in balancing itself and increasing energy.

LINK #14

EMOTIONAL RESCUE FOR YOU!:
BACH FLOWER REMEDIES

Ever feel like you're having difficulty with balancing out your emotions, are you in a pattern of negative repetition and nothing seems to work? You're on a merry-go-round of what seems like craziness? It is also possible that you're not aware of certain patterns that you repeat that others are constantly reminding you of and you don't see or understand what they are talking about.

Bach Flowers to the RESCUE!!! I LOVE Bach Flowers! I use them and have suggested these essences to clients who have hit a plateau in their wellness program. They are also great to incorporate at the beginning and during a program to assist with many negative emotions such as:

- ADD, ADHD
- Anger
- Anxiety
- Control Issues
- Daydreaming
- Depression
- Emotional Eating
- Fear
- Hate
- Inability to Focus
- increasing confidence
- Insomnia
- Panic Attacks
- Passive
- Resentment
- Self-Absorption
- Stress
- Trauma

- Weight Issues
- And many more negative emotions and issues

Dr. Edward Bach created Bach Flower Remedies in England nearly 100 years ago. There are 38 single remedies and 1 combination remedy that are used to remove negative emotions and replace them with the positive energy.

BACH FLOWER REMEDIES:

1. *Agrimony* – helps those who tend to hold their feelings inside and tend to rely on substances such as drugs and alcohol to cope. They keep a smile on their face even when they feel tortured internally. Use of this essence allows a person to realize that it's not necessary to always be happy and it's okay to be sad or show other emotions sometimes.

   Persons with this type of personality are likely to suffer from disorders such as hypo- or hypertension, drug and/or alcohol addictions, hair loss, premature graying.

2. *Aspen* – This helps those who are constantly in a state of fear. These fears may originate from a traumatic event such as abuse, rape, being afraid of the dark or some other trauma. This essence gives a person the strength to face their fears.

   This personality type may have problems with acne, incontinence, rapid heartbeat, phobias and hypertension.

3. *Beech* – Helps those who tend to have very rigid ideas and standards, are unwilling to bend and consider others thoughts and suggestions. They tend to think everyone should only follow them without question and does not easily accept others opinions. They are perfectionists and expecting others to always do more, be better, never apologize or admit fault. Their nature is to be bossy, ambitious and aggressive.

Physical problems this personality is likely to suffer include hypertension, fatigue, indigestion, headache and irritability.

4. *Centaury* – Is for those who are shy, timid and don't know how to say "no". They are always willing to sacrifice their needs for others regardless how it may affect them. Tends to not offer their opinion, love peace, and are often taken advantage of by others.

    They may suffer from malnutrition, anemia, low blood pressure, pains in the joints, or low blood sugar issues.

5. *Cetero* – Helps those who are inconsistent in their thinking and doing, has a hard time making decisions, impatient, does not trust their own decisions but does not trust others even when seeking advice from them, lacks confidence, inability to stick to a regimen for an extended period of time.

    Health problems experienced may include high or low blood pressure, migraines, ulcers.

6. Cherry Plum – Aids those who are afraid they will "lose it" and want to explode and not be able to control themselves and emotions. Has tendency towards potentially harming themselves and others through violent actions.
    This personality may experience issues such as high blood pressure, eating disorders, heart palpitations and heart rate, and anger problems.

7. *Chestnut* Bud – Beneficial to those who do not learn from the past and continue to make same mistakes over and over even when they are aware of them, have and very happy about life attitude.

    Any physical problems associated with this type of personality are individual and have to be evaluated that way.

8. *Chicory* – Helps those who tend to be overly possessive but are also loving and kind, will do whatever they think necessary to win your affections even if in a manipulative manner. They expect to be rewarded for whatever favors or duties they do for you in order to get something in return.

   This personality type tends to suffer from issues such as: weakness, high blood pressure highs and lows, hair loss, irritability, eating disorders.

9. *Clematis* – Helps those who tend to be daydreamers – are constantly "in their heads", not happy or satisfied with their lives, can be somewhat antisocial, has difficulty concentrating, not very attentive or interested in what's going on around them.

   Issues with this personality can lead to psychological problems it left untreated for long time; also tend to be clumsy and careless, may experience falls, anemia, malnutrition and weakness.

10. *Crab Apple* – Helps those who don't feel like they're clean or physically attractive. Obsess over small things and overlook those things that matter. May be depressed and suffer from low self-esteem.

    Symptoms that may appear in this personality type include lack of confidence, anxiety, nausea and vomiting, irritability and tendency to become overexcited.

11. *Elm* – Helps these good-natured, hard-working, responsible focused individuals keep up their confidence when stressed, anxious or overworked stay on track.

    Problems associated with this personality type includes stomach problems, headaches including migraines and unstable blood pressure.

12. *Gentian* – Helps those who allow even in small setbacks or problems to get to them, and are easily discouraged. They are often negative and skeptical when faced with hard times and difficult situations. Always feel like they are under pressure and are very tense.

This personality type tends to suffer from high cholesterol, constipation and diarrhea, ulcers, high blood pressure, and headaches.

13. *Gorse* – Helps those you have feelings of great hopelessness and have given up on believing that anything can change for them. If persuaded, may try something different, while at the same time convincing others that there is little hope that things will get better.

This personality may suffer from hair loss, weakness, dizziness, headaches, weight loss, dry lips, and headaches.

14. *Heather* – Helps those who tend to be self-centered, loves to be the center of attention as much as possible, only concerned about what's going on with them, will share their problems with anyone who will listen. Tend to be possessive, focused attention seekers.

This personality type suffers from problems with eating disorders and blood pressure.

15. *Holly* – Helps those who tend to be jealous, vengeful, antisocial, greedy, cold-hearted, egotistic, short-tempered and controlling. They have problems with internal emotional trauma possibly due to constantly comparing themselves to others and not accepting others as they are.

Other problems they may suffer include heart, blood pressure and skin issues.

16. _Honeysuckle_ – Helps those who tend to live in the past, not looking at what's good in their present situation. Tend to become homesick, longing for the "good old days" when things where better. Has difficulty adjusting to new situations and environments.

   This personality suffers from depression, anemia, anxiety, irritability, short temper, anxiety and irritability.

17. _Hornbeam_ – Helps those who know how or what needs to be accomplished but are afraid or have difficulty getting started. They just need a push or encouragement to begin. Once started are able to complete what they set out to do.

   This personality type often deals with constipation and other bowel problems, eating disorders, unstable blood pressure, frequent urination, heart palpitations, and sweating.

18. _Impatiens_ -- As the word indicates, this helps those who are impatient with others and processes that take more time than they feel it should. Would rather do things for and by themselves so that they can do things at their own speed and pace because their mind is quick and they want things done right away.

   This personality type may have problems with sleep, hypertension and ulcers.

19. _Larch_ – Helps those who are not confident in their own abilities, but genuinely and easily praises and supports accomplishments of others. Refuses to compete with others because they believe they will fail or cannot win. Can become depressed and lack self-esteem.

   This personality type may suffer from hair loss, dry lips, pale skin, circles under the eyes and weakness.

20. *Mimilus* – Helps those who are very sensitive, easily embarrassed and nervous. Helps with overcoming fears such as being alone, spiders, losing work, pain. They try to hide these fears from others.

Problems that may present with this personality type include fainting, tremors, bedwetting, and talk that doesn't seem relevant at the time.

21. *Mustard* – This helps when one experiences sudden depression without a reason. Such as a dark cloud that takes away any happiness, then lifts all of a sudden just as it came.

This personality type may suffer from low blood pressure, anorexia, sleep problems, hair loss, dry lips, extreme irritability and dark circles under eyes.

22. *Oak* -- Helps when overworked and are an over-achiever and will go beyond fatigue to accomplish. They did not give up even under most difficult situations and do not like to be reminded they should slow down or get rest. They are mentally, physically and emotionally ready to deal with the most difficult situations and not give up or give in.

With this personality type, it is difficult to know when they are having health concerns because they will not easily acknowledge them easily.

23. *Olive* – Helps those who are dealing with physical exhaustion or when a person has no energy, is tired, feels faint or restless. Also helps when one is just overcoming serious illness or emotional trauma.

This personality type may suffer from fatigue, dizziness, weakness and fatigue.

24. *Pine* – Helps those who are never satisfied with their accomplishments. Even when taking credit for what they accomplished will blame themselves for everything that may have gone wrong. Although hard working and patient, have problems with self -esteem because they don't appreciate or value themselves.

Symptoms they may display include asthma, blood pressure highs and lows, headaches and problems with skin.

25. Red Chestnut – Assists those who worry and are concerned about other problems in an overwhelming way that causes them to become disturbed and distressed. They are very open-hearted, loving and are overly subtle and tend to over think things which only causes them more anxiety and stress.

Problems they are likely to suffer include dry lips, hair loss, blood pressure highs and lows, allergies, asthma, low weight issues, and circles under eyes.

26. Rescue Remedy – This is a combination of 5 Bach Flowers (Cherry Plum, Clematis, Impatiens, Rock Rose and Star of Bethlehem). Helps in times of stress when keeping emotions in check is imperative such as in the case of medical or emotional emergencies, trauma to help calm nerves and spirit (does not take the place of medical assistance).

Problems associated with this personality are blood sugar imbalances, fainting, tremors, blood pressure highs and lows and heart palpitations.

27. Rock Rose -- Helps those who feel unclear and can't move forward due to fright and terror. They are afraid to face situations that may be scary or traumatic, so they carry this fear even when there is nothing to fear. This may cause nightmares, extreme worry and shock.

This personality type may suffer from problems with sleep including sleep walking and eating disorders.

28. _Rose Water_ – Helps those with very high ambitions and goals, have big egos, and tend to be self-centered. They work very hard to accomplish any goals they set for themselves, are very confident but are not very flexible.

This personality type takes great care of themselves so are not sick very often but if they are it is from overworking and exertion.

29. _Sclerantus_ – Helps those who have hard time making decisions, are inconsistent in their actions, confused about what to do and have difficulty sharing what's going on with them with others.

This personality tends to experience tremors, slurred or difficulty speech, and motion sickness.

30. _Star of Bethlehem_ – Helps those who may be recovering from some type of emotional trauma or shock but are equipped to handle the situation. However, the results of the shock and trauma has been set and must be removed and eliminated.

This personality type has a tendency towards problems with metabolism, blood pressure issues (high and low), skin and headaches.

31. _Sweet Chestnut_ – Helps for those who have reached their limit and they have come to a point where they cannot move forward. Physical and mental limits have been reached and can't take anymore.

Health problems they may experience include hair loss, blood pressure issues, stomach problems, nausea, dizziness, eating disorders.

32. _Vervain_ – Helps those with very strong will power, are ambitious, extremely hardworking but sensitive, puts on a brave face no matter what they are going through.

This personality type tends to have issues in these areas: skin problems, hormonal, blood pressure and blood sugar imbalances, and pain in joints.

33. _Vine_ – Helps those who are extremely egoistical, domineering, are very confident, dictators – their way or the highway! They know everything even if they have to mix some "untruths" in their opinions. This personality type is not very flexible or open to the viewpoints of others.

It's difficult for them to admit when something is wrong with them because they are not the "problem" but the "solution" to everything.

34. _Walnut_ – Helps those who are having difficulty adjusting to changes in their life, whether it be moving to a new location, breakup in a relationship, a new job, etc.

This personality type may experience problems with sinuses, allergies and mood changes.

35. _Water Violet_ – Helps those who are loners and are aware of the fact that they feel superior to others, prefer to deal with their problems on their own without the help of others. They tend to be very independent whether on their own or in a group.

Physical problems this personality type may suffer include lowered immune system, anemia, headaches including migraines, weakness, low energy, and problems sleeping.

36. _White Chestnut_ – Helps those who are unable to make decisions because they are always in their thoughts about how to juggle

several decisions at once. Unable to sleep due to thoughts that clutter the mind.

This personality type tends to suffer from these physical issues: stomach problems, irritability, headaches, fatigue, easily upset, and circles under the eyes.

37. _Wild Oat_ – Helps those who tend to lack direction, because of their intelligence, hard work ethic and ability to easily excel in several different areas, are unable to choose and focus on any one area. They lack good time management skills because of their inability to concentrate on anything long enough to see progress in a chosen field.

The personality type may have problems with malnutrition, hair loss, irritability, weight loss or eating disorders.

38. _Wild Rose_ -- Helps those who feel like giving up and can't see things getting better, can't seem to find solution to all that they have suffered. They have lost the excitement in life, appear emotionless, stagnant and unwilling to seek help.

This personality type tends to suffer these physical problems: muscle mass loss, anemia, hair loss, and malnutrition.

39. _Willow_ -- Helps after having suffered an adversity and misfortune that is difficult to face. Having a "poor me" attitude, blames others for their misfortunes. Comes off as being ungrateful and unappreciative.

Physical problems with this personality type may include heart issues, skin problems, blood pressure highs and lows, heart problems.

As you can see Bach Flowers covered a myriad of emotional and mental concerns. This listing is only a brief summary of how these wonderful remedies can be used to help bring about emotional and mental stability unconsciously. They can also be used on pets and plants!

LINK #15

POUR A L'IL OIL ON ME!: USE OF AROMATHERAPY AND ESSENTIAL OILS

Aromatherapy is a holistic treatment based on the external use (sometimes internal) of essential aromatic plant oils to maintain and promote physical, physiological, and spiritual wellbeing. The essential oils may be used in massage, added to a warm bath, used to moisten a compress that is applied to a particular affected part of the body, added to a vaporizer for inhalation or diffused throughout a room to freshen and even disinfect and many other uses.

ESSENTIAL OILS ARE:
- Subtle, volatile liquids distilled from plants, shrubs, flowers, trees, roots, bushes and seeds.
- Chemically, very complex, consisting of hundreds of chemical compounds.
- The most powerful part of the plant.
- Closely linked to physical, emotional and spiritual wellbeing.
- Used to kill bacteria, fungi, viruses, fight infection

Human blood and the essential oils of plants share several common properties. Both start the process of regeneration of cells, fight infection and contain hormone-like properties. The distilling of an ENTIRE plant may only produce a SINGLE DROP of essential oil.

ESSENTIAL OILS CAN:
- Helps with mood
- Lifts spirits
- Dispel negative emotions
- Create romantic atmosphere
- Stimulates regeneration of tissues and

- Oxygenates nerves
- Carry nutrients to cells

HOW TO USE ESSENTIAL OILS:
- Most essential oils should be mixed with a carrier oil such as grapeseed, jojoba (pronounced ho-ho-ba), almond, etc. due to potency on skin
- Peppermint and lavender can be applied directly on the skin without using a carrier oil
- In a diffuser, mix with water as a spray, inhaled, ingested or applied topically.
- Can be used in massage, reflexology, acupuncture, and other forms of bodywork and treatments.
- Many oils CANNOT be used during pregnancy so consult with a professional who is proficient in use of essential oils

COMMON ESSENTIAL OILS
and THEIR POTENTIAL EFFECTS:

Peppermint – *antifungal, antibacterial, stimulant, supports digestion, heighten or restore sense of taste.*

Lavender – calming, relaxing, balancing, antiseptic, analgesic (pain), cleaning cuts, burns (cell renewal), headaches.

Tea Tree – antifungal, antiviral, antiseptic, immune-stimulant, anti-inflammatory, anti-bacterial.

Eucalyptus – analgesic, antiviral, antibacterial, insect repellent, antifungal, sores, wounds.

Jasmine – uplifting and stimulating, reduces anxiety, increases excitability when worn as fragrance.

Patchouli – beneficial to skin, prevents wrinkles or chapped skin, sedating, calming, relaxing, antimicrobial, antiseptic, helps itching.

BIBLICAL OILS

Frankincense – Increases spiritual awareness and promotes meditation, help improve attitude, uplift spirits, strengthen immune system.

Myrrh – Promotes spiritual awareness and is uplifting, anti-infectious, antiviral, supports immune system, candida, fungal infection, gum infections, gingivitis.

Cinnamon – Antimicrobial anti-infectious, antiviral, antifungal, sexual stimulant, beneficial for circulation.

Essential Oils that Affect the Liver and Lymphatic System

Geranium – dilates bile ducts for liver detoxification

Rosemary – hepatitis

Roman chamomile – cleanses blood, helps liver discharge poisons, promotes digestion, reduces indigestion

German chamomile – cleanses blood, helps liver function and secretion, supports the pancreas

The following combination cleanses the liver and the lymphatic system of high levels of toxins. It assists in the process of breaking up any anger and hate stored in the liver. Apply over liver, solar plexus or use as in a whole body massage.

Juniper Berry – This powerful, detoxifying oil is a purifier, helps avert nervous tension, and reduces cellulite. Juniper essential oil is an antiviral, antiseptic, diuretic and can help relieve pain, the symptoms of rheumatism, and expel uric acid from the system. Juniper's spicy aroma helps to strengthen and fortify the spirit during times of low energy, anxiety, and emotional overload. The oil can irritate some people's skin and should be avoided during pregnancy.

Helichrysum – Ideal for use during a drug or alcohol detox, helichrysum helps stimulate liver cells, thin mucous secretion, and acts as a free radical scavenger. It Is non-toxic and non-irritating.

Lemon – A refreshing citrus oil, lemon stimulates white blood cells to defend the body against infection. Its detoxifying and regenerating properties are beneficial for the liver, and aid in bring clarity to the mind and emotions. Lemon may irritate those with sensitive skin and when used in a bath it must be used with a carrier oil.

Grapefruit – Having a detoxifying effect on individuals recovering from substance abuse, grapefruit is antiviral, antiseptic, diuretic, and can aid the digestive system and skin. It refreshes the mind, relieves anxiety, is reviving, uplifting, and helps disperse negative energy. It may, however, increase photosensitivity.

Essential oils are an easy and effective way to build the immune system, eliminate pain and has so many other healing properties that definitely should be a part of your health regimen. As with any other product, choose high quality oils.

LINK #16

IT'S ALL IN YOUR HAND – AND FEET
BENEFITS OF REFLEXOLOGY

As a Reflexologist, I have had the pleasure and opportunity to assist many people benefit from the use of this wonderful and powerful form of bodywork.

Exactly what is reflexology? According to Dwight C. Byers, author of *"Better Health with Reflexology, The Ingham Method*, it is defined as "a science that deals with the principle that there are reflex areas in the feet and hands that correspond to all the glands, organs and parts of the body. Reflexology is a unique method of using the thumbs and fingers in these reflex areas.

Although reflexology is becoming a better known holistic health technique, it had not always been a common choice in today's world. The use of reflexology goes back over 2,000 years to ancient Egypt. There is are writings that were found on the tomb of a physician that translates as "Don't hurt me" with the reply from the practitioner of "I shall act so you praise me." It shows that the act of this technique will bring about pleasure to the person receiving the treatment. I don't look for praise for myself but for the satisfaction that my client receives the benefits that this process provides.

Most people are aware of foot reflexology, however, there are different types of reflexology including, hand, ear, facial and body reflexology. God, in His glory and grace, created the human body to be pretty much self-contained in the sense that almost everything we need to help heal us is within us. There are 10 zones or meridians that extend from the hands, feet, throughout the body and the head. By pressing on the hands and/or feet on different parts, one can help bring relief to every organ, body part and system within that "zone".

There are studies that have shown the benefits of reflexology way beyond that of just relaxation. Studies prove the use of this treatment has positive effect on all kinds of illnesses and diseases.

The simple act of touch has been found to be relaxing and reduces tension for both the giver and receiver. Studies have shown that "the stimulation of reflexology's pressure techniques creates change in our body's basic level of tension as demonstrated by research using measurement of brain waves (EEG), blood pressure, systolic blood pressure, diastolic blood pressure, pulse rate, and anxiety. One study of a single session noted that reflexology has a ".....powerful anxiety-reduction effect."

Here are a few techniques you can use on yourself or loved ones:

Arthritis
Grab and squeeze the meaty part of the hand between the thumb and index finger. Hold and squeeze for several minutes. Do on both hands. Also press the padding on the palm side of the hands just below the finger joints and above the palms of the hands. Work from index finger side to baby finger side several times.

This helps increase circulation, releases toxins and decreases inflammation. (can work referral areas if areas are too tender)

BODY SYSTEMS AFFECTED: Adrenals, liver, kidneys, lymph nodes

Asthma
Press the padding on the hands just below the finger joints and above the palm of the hands. Work from index finger side to baby finger side several times. On the back side of the hand, use the thumb of the opposite hand, and press between the spaces of each finger down to the middle of the back of the hand.

Can relieve tension and decrease inflammation of bronchial passages, reduce infection.

Stimulates the solar plexus, diaphragm, lungs spine, adrenals, and other upper body points

Back Pain
Press and hold the area below the bony part of palm between the index and middle fingers, also "walk" up and down from the bottom of heel of hand up to top of thumb and reverse.

Helps open up energy flow to brain, reduces pain

BODY SYSTEMS AFFECTED: spine, upper and lower back, increase circulation and blood flow

Constipation/Gas/Flatulence
Sit on the toilet with right hand on thigh with palm up, take opposite elbow and press and rub in circular motion into center of hand; reverse.

Helps open up bowel flow to stimulate and increase evacuation and relieve gas.

BODY SYSTEMS AFFECTED: colon, liver, gallbladder, stomach

Fatigue
Using 2 or 3 fingers together and tap the center of chest and/or press tongue on roof of mouth just in front of teeth. Do this for 1-2 minutes.

Increases and opens up energy and reduces fatigue.

BODY SYSTEM AFFECTED: Thymus

Headache
Press tips and sides of fingers on both hands. Find tender spots and concentrate on these areas until headache subsides.

Reduces or eliminates pain, increases circulation in head.

BODY SYSTEMS AFFECTED: Head, spine, neck, shoulders, adrenals

Menopausal/PMS
Press around the wrist area on both sides of the arm as well as up the inside of arm towards the elbows.

BODY SYSTEMS AFFECTED: Ovary/Testicle, Uterus/Prostate, lower back

Pain
Press and hold the meaty part of the hand between the thumb and index finger. Hold for several minutes. Do on both hands.

Reduces or eliminates pain in affected body part.

BODY SYSTEMS AFFECTED: Depends on body part affected, including adrenals, circulation.

Sciatica
Lay hands crisscross one another palms together, take fingers of bottom hand and press into top of hand on top near wrist.

Opens up circulation in back of legs, lower back and pelvic area.

BODY SYSTEMS AFFECTED: Legs, lower back, pelvic, sciatic nerve, hip

These simple, self-help tips can be used between receiving hand or foot reflexology from a professional. They are helpful, but if you have never tried reflexology, you owe it to yourself to get a session scheduled as soon as possible!! You'll love it!!

CONCLUSION

In the first edition of the book, *"10 Tips to Strengthen Your Body's Weakest Links"* my goal was to give you information that I had gathered from presentations from my seminar entitled *"What's Your Body's Weakest Link"*. In this revised version, I have expanded and added additional links that I believe are essential to helping you achieve wellness at a higher level. My intention for writing this book is to provide suggestions that can be easily introduced into your health lifestyle as well as introduce some thoughts about your body functions that will help make sense of the importance of keeping your temple and your SOUL functioning at its highest peak.

In the introduction of the first edition, *"10 Tips to Strengthen Your Body's Weakest Links"*, I gave a brief overview of my journey to wellness. I mentioned this journey began with a series of health issues that started in my mid-teens and persisted into my forties. Even though I feel I have recovered from the serious symptoms, episodes and issues I dealt with during those years, each day is a test and testament of the ups, downs, successes and disappointments I have experienced. Over the past 10-15 years I have dealt with weight, hormonal, emotional and still some physical problems as I mature into my senior years.

Overall I feel that my maturing years have been very good _to_ me and _for_ me. Yes, I have grown mentally, emotionally......yes, even physically! Dealing with serious health concerns from my youth into middle age and then being blessed to have recovered to a point that not even I could have imagined, has given me the opportunity to come to a better understanding of how my body works. Because of this I have a perspective that I believe is almost necessary in order to have insight into the problems and concerns my clients and others have. I stress to my clients that being in tuned to their body's reactions, feelings and quirks is the first key to maintaining their health.

No one is as close to you as YOU are. Listen to and respect the "signals" your body gives you. I'm not saying that every little twitch or pain is a sign of something serious going on. However, if that twitch or pain persists over a time that's unusual and not normal, don't ignore it! Seek help from your medical doctor or health care professional.

I am often asked how did I get started in the natural health field? I would say that it began long before I realized it. I recall during my early teen years I began to experience various problems with my health. I had some vision, digestive including constipation as well as some balance problems.

One particular incident which stands out was at the age of 16, while simply walking through the house I fell – just hit the floor for what seemed to be no apparent reason. I was unable to move or get up off the floor. I was taken to the hospital where the only problem found was that I was anemic. Of course, I was prescribed iron tablets, this only added to my problems of constipation! Uugggh!!

Over the next 10-15 years I endured many health problems and was unable to get clear answers to the symptoms and complaints I was experiencing. I went to several different medical specialists, including psychiatrist *("it's all in your head, young lady!")*, otolaryngologists *("you just have a sinus infection!")*, an orthopedic doctor *("we can't find anything wrong, try physical therapy")* and other medical professionals but ultimately there was no real solution to my problems.

I eventually went to a neurologist. Initially, I was told that I had some "demyelization" in my spine but it was something I didn't have to worry about until I was much older. So of course, I didn't put much thought into that, I was only in my mid-20's at that time. "Older" was something in the very distant future, my concern was for my very present situation.

Finally, around the age of 30, after my symptoms were getting continually worse, I went back to the neurologist and after many tests – all of which came back negative, I was eventually diagnosed with Multiple Sclerosis (MS), a disease of the central nervous system.

This puzzled me because none of the test showed any plaques on my spine or brain. So I questioned the doctor how could he diagnose me with MS when all tests came back "normal". His answer was that I fell in that 10% of people where tests don't show anything and he based his diagnosis on "classic" MS symptoms.

It was true I displayed all the typical signs of MS: vision problems, extreme fatigue, balance problems, numbness and tingling in feet and hands, slurred speech, sometimes inability to talk or walk at all, paralysis, spastic colon, spasms, jerky body movements (ataxia), incontinence, memory problems, inability to connect my thoughts to action and other symptoms that are considered typical of MS.

Over the years my problems became progressively worse until I was experiencing difficulty walking without the assistance of a cane or walker as well as times when I could not walk at all. Even though I was not given a diagnosis until this time, my problems may have actually began with that first fall at the age of 16.

I tried the typical regimen with traditional medicine – taking prescription medications, steroid IV's, and all kinds of tests, but I only became worse. I reacted to every medication I was given, even had an experience with an IV steroid that sent me into convulsions and possible anaphylactic shock.

Then in 1995 I was introduced to a couple named Greg (may he rest in peace) and his wife, Erin Taylor who owned a natural health store called The Herbalist in Cincinnati, Ohio. Erin who at the time was a Master Herbalist and eventually become a holistic naturopath, suggested an herbal regimen that I followed EXACTLY according to her suggestions, in addition to the dietary and other changes I had already implemented.

Over time I began to see positive changes in my health. The improvement was by no means overnight, but with persistence and consistency, I was able to turn my health around 180 degrees! It was still a long, hard road but I was DETERMINED to change my health condition. I KNOW my faith in God had a lot to do with it – no, let me rephrase that – it had EVERYTHING to do with it!

I trusted and believed that I would get better. I prayed every day that one day I would be able to run again (something I would do before my health took a downward turn). It was 15 years before I realized that I could run again.

We ask God to help us with a problem we are going through and need help to overcome, and then we put conditions, deadlines and scenarios on how we want Him to resolve them. By this I mean, we pray, shout, plead and ask for something to change or be fixed by this time or that time and that it should come in the way, shape, form and the timing we want or think it to be. When it doesn't happen, we think He has abandoned us or has not heard us. It could be that He has already answered your prayer but we don't notice because it doesn't look, sound, smell or taste the way we thought it should be or in the form or person we want it to be.

For me, I just prayed no matter what, in fact, the day I found out I could run, I didn't realize it until I was told that I had just ran. I had started an MS support group and one day while crossing the street to attend the meeting, I ran across the street because I was a little late, some of the members were looking out the window and saw me. When I entered the building, everyone was crying tears of joy and happiness while shouting out to me "You ran, you ran!" I just looked bewildered and said "What?" I didn't know that I had ran!! Had I not already shared my prayer with them, seeing me run would not have been such a big deal and I would not have known that God had already answered my prayer.

That was 15 years after I began asking for this miracle! Is it possible that I had ran long before that? I say that I probably did, but only because the members in the support group knew my story and was able to tell me. Otherwise, I would not have paid much attention to the fact that I could run. I believe because I was not putting a timeline on God doing His work, I trusted and He made it happen for me – in His timing and according to HIS plan and obviously without my input!

Over the years I found not only was my central nervous system very weak, but I also suffered from extreme hypoglycemia, sometimes walking around with a blood sugar level of 30 (the low end of normal is 70) as well as suffering from extreme pernicious anemia (inability to absorb iron). Many of the symptoms of these two dis-eases are similar to those of multiple sclerosis. These two ailments went untreated for years because the focus was only directed at the neurological symptoms.

A third issue was brought to my attention by The Herbalist team – the amalgam (mercury) fillings in my teeth. I had 8 teeth that had mercury fillings in them. As a person who has to understand the "why" of things, I did my research on mercury/amalgam fillings. I spent 9 months reading everything – positive and negative – about the effects of mercury fillings and how to safely have them replaced.

I requested and had blood tests done to determine levels of heavy metals in my system. My doctor ordered blood work through the local labs. Guess what? Yes, the lab work came back NORMAL!! Surprise! Surprise!! No heavy metals were detected in my blood. In spite of this, I was not satisfied that this was true.

I finally consulted with 2 biological dentists to find out the process and safety of having the fillings removed and what would be used to replace them. Both were excellent dentists and found I had high levels of mercury in my teeth and body.

The first dentist used a type of machine that measured the levels of mercury in each tooth. Each time the pointer would fly to the extreme end of the chart. The second dentist used kinesiology (muscle testing) and liquid drops of different heavy metals under my tongue to determine my sensitivity to each of the metals.

I chose to go to the second dentist because I was familiar with kinesiology/muscle testing. When he put the drops of each heavy metal under my tongue, I reacted negatively to all of them. However, when he put the mercury under my tongue, within 15-20 seconds, I began to respond by convulsing violently and nearly coming out of the chair. Even the dentist was surprised by how strongly I reacted to the mercury.

So, needless to say, I was convinced I had to have those fillings removed and replaced. Even though I had made drastic changes to my diet, lifestyle by reducing stress, getting proper rest, sticking to the suggested herbal regimen, etc., once I had the mercury fillings removed, my life and health took a drastic change for the better within less than 3 months. I was on a detox regimen specifically for helping to remove the heavy metals, especially the mercury from my teeth as well as from my body on a cellular level.

Over time my health continued to improve. Previously, I had only been able to work about 20 hours a week. By the end of 3 months I was able to go back to work full time. Something I had not been able to do for several years!

What I found was that many of the symptoms of MS, anemia, hypoglycemia and mercury poisoning have overlapping, common characteristics *(see chart at back of book)*. Once I was able to correct these problems, I no longer had to rely on a cane, I was able to work without staggering and I live a fairly normal life now. When I meet people now they would have no idea the journey I have been through. What a blessing!

I am not a medical doctor (and I don't play one on TV!), however, I don't believe what I experienced was truly multiple sclerosis. Over the years I have and continue to work on improving my health. Excellent health is not something you get and then you're done. It's a way of life and has to periodically be adjusted depending on lifestyle, diet, hormonal changes, genetics, environment, emotions, stress, age and other factors.

Getting through this journey was not easy. Sometimes I wonder how did I make it without losing my mind. A lot of it was having a sense of humor and not always taking everything too seriously while at the same time recognizing how SERIOUS things really were.

Growing up I watched my mother deal with severe physical health problems. When I was about 5 years old she broke her back in a bus accident. I recall her being on a walker and wearing a back brace for what seemed like years. Doctors said she would not walk again and would be paralyzed. But she said NO! She was determined she would walk again and SHE DID!!

I know I got my tenacity from her! SHE NEVER GAVE UP!! In fact, she became pregnant with our youngest brother while she was in that back brace!! After I was grown, married and had a child of my own, I got up the nerves to ask her how did that happen? Well.....I won't tell you what she said, but suffice it to say that all I could say was -- oookkkaaay!! Then I let it go! Mom had a great sense of humor in dealing with her health issues.

It's important to know how _your_ body and body systems respond to inside and outside stimuli. When upset, does your stomach become tied in knots? Do you get a headache? Do you become depressed? Do your shoulders tense up? Being aware of _YOUR_ unique body is the key to determining YOUR body's weakest link — and coming up with a plan to strengthen it, as well as keeping the ones that are not weak – remain STRONG!

I have found that my central nervous system is my body's weakest link as well as my digestive system, particularly, my liver. It was this journey of wellness that led me to discovering how my body responds to the lifestyle choices I made – positive and negative -- over the years.

I don't believe my health problems are anything special or more outstanding than anyone else who is going through or has gone through trials and tribulations – this is just MY story. I share it so that others can be inspired and hopefully seek ways to improve their health and know that they are not alone in overcoming obstacles in their lives. I hope you found this book a simple, easy read that will assist you on your health journey.

COMPARISON OF SYMPTOMS CHART

Multiple Sclerosis	Hypoglycemia (low blood sugar)	Mercury Poisoning	Pernicious Anemia
Bladder problems	Dizziness	Chronic diarrhea/ constipation	Urinary incontinence
Bowel problems	Inappropriate behavior or severe confusion	Cognitive decline	Fecal incontinence
Breathing problems	Fatigue	Mental depression, despondency	Depression
Cognitive changes	Headache	Dizziness/acute, chronic vertigo	Dizziness
Depression	Heart Palpitations	Emotional instability	Confusion
Dizziness and Vertigo	Hunger	Fatigue	Fatigue
Emotional changes	Lightheadedness	Chronic headaches	Memory loss; impaired memory
Fatigue	Nervousness	Abnormal heart rhythm	Numbness and tingling in hands and feet
Headache	Tingling feeling around mouth	Loss of memory	Spasticity
Hearing Loss	Seizures	Numbness and tingling of hands, feet, fingers, toes, or lips	Difficulty walking
Itching	Slurred speech	Twitching	Lack of coordination, clumsiness
Numbness and Tingling	Shakiness	Speech problems	Incoordination
Seizures	Visual disturbances	Tremors/trembling of hands, feet, lips, eyelids or tongue	Weight loss
Sexual problems	Unsteadiness when standing or walking	Visual impairment, Glaucoma, Restricted, dim vision	Shortness of breath
Spasticity	Weakness	Difficulty walking	

117

Multiple Sclerosis	Hypoglycemia (low blood sugar)	Mercury Poisoning	Pernicious Anemia
Speech problems	Clumsiness	Muscle weakness progressing to paralysis	
Swallowing problems	Inability to concentrate	Inability to concentrate	
Tremor	Unconsciousness	Lethargy/drowsiness	
Vision problems	Poor control of movements	Shyness or timidity, being easily embarrassed	
Walking (gait) difficulties	Irritability	Exaggerated response to Stimulation	
Weakness	Anxiety	Indecision	
	Crying out during sleep	Loss of self confidence	
	Loss of consciousness	Fearfulness	
		Ataxia	
		Bleeding gums	
		Loosening of teeth	
		Metallic taste	
		Allergies	
		Burning sensation, with tingling of lips face	
		Ringing in the ears	
		Hearing difficulties	
		Abnormal blood pressure (either high or low)	
		Food sensitivities, esp. to milk and eggs	
		Abdominal cramps, colitis, diverticulitis or other G.I. complaint Unexplained reactivity	
		Hypoglycemia	
		Loss of weight	

Multiple Sclerosis	Hypoglycemia (low blood sugar)	Mercury Poisoning	Pernicious Anemia
		Loss of appetite, with or without weight loss	
		Repeated infections: Viral and fungal Mycobacteria Candida and other yeast infections	
		General fatigue	
		Unexplained sensory symptoms, including pain	
		Cold clammy skin esp. hands and feet	
		Thyroid disturbance	
		Unexplained anemia	
		Unexplained numbness or burning sensations	
		Subnormal body temperature	
		Physical discomfort	
		Tissue pigmentation (amalgam tattoo of gums)	
		Ulceration of gingiva, palate, tongue	
		Multiple sclerosis	

SUMMARY

The information in this book is not intended to replace your health care professional or medical doctor. It is simply meant to help you gain an understanding of how YOU have control over your life and health – not just a longer life, but one of quality, goodness and happiness.

It provides strategies to a holistic, balanced life and *discovering your body's weakest link* and some possible solutions to make your body and SOUL strong and healthy. Each of the topics discussed can be considered separately or in combination with others to obtain some results.

You are not alone in this journey, I am here to support you and direct you in reaching your goals and providing information that will allow you to make conscious, easy-to-follow steps toward wellness.

My goal is to help as many people as I can to be the BEST they can be with what God has given them. Through my own trials and tribulations, I have found that if I put my trust in God and I mean TRULY – LET GO AND LET GOD! that He will quickly take care of my needs. However, in the meantime, we must keep walking toward our goals so that at the end of the road you will find that it will work out BETTER than you could have ever imagined!

Remember: You are "wonderfully and fearfully made!" There is no one on this earth EXACTLY like YOU! Your uniqueness is special, so EMBRACE YOUR SOUL! – exactly as it is TODAY and move forward as you make changes to improve and strengthen your body's weakest link(s).

Now that you have read all the way through, take a few minutes to write down 2 to 3 of the Links that you would like to utilize within the next few days. Put them in the order of importance to you and apply them over the next few weeks or months. Keep a journal to track your feelings, progress and any thoughts or reactions you experience.

Feel free to send any questions you may have using my contact information below.

Be patient, kind, loving and accepting of where you are RIGHT NOW. When you backslide, forget or just plain don't want to do anything, just pick up from where you are and KEEP ON STEPPING and HEAL THY SOUL!!!

With Love and Care,

Roberta T. McClinon

Author
Naturopathic and Holistic Health Consultant
Registered Certified Reflexologist
Reiki II Practitioner
Internet Radio Host
docro@healthysoulstherapy.com
www.healthysoulstherapy.com
www.blogtalkradio.com/healthy-soul-talk

GLOSSARY

Adrenal Stimulant -- Substance increases the action of the adrenal glands

Analgesic -- May relieve pain

Anesthetic -- May relieve pain

Anodyne -- May relieve pain

Antibacterial -- Substance that may potentially destroy or stop bacterial infection growth

Anticoagulant -- Substance that thins blood and may prevent clotting

Anti-carcinogen – Substance that fights against cancer

Antidepressant -- Substance that may relieve depression symptoms

Antifungal -- Substance that may destroy or prevent fungus growth

Antihistamine -- Substance may neutralize histamine effect in an allergic response

Anti-inflammatory -- Substance that may reduce the effects of inflammation

Antimicrobial -- Substance that may destroy or prevent growth of microorganisms

Anti-neoplastic -- Substance that may prevent malignant cell growth

Antioxidant -- Keeps free radicals or oxidation from damaging tissues and cells

Antiparasitic – Substance that kills parasites

Antispasmodic -- Agent that prevents or relieves spasms

Antiviral -- Opposing the action of a virus

Aromatic -- Agent that contains volatile essential oils which aids digestion and relieves gas

Astringent – Agent that has binding and constricting properties

Carminative -- Relieves intestinal gas and distension; promotes peristalsis (bowel action)

Digestive stimulant -- Aids digestions, usually by providing enzymes from various sources

Diaphoretic -- Agent that causes perspiration and increases elimination through skin

Diuretic -- Increases the secretion and flow of urine

Expectorant -- Encourages the loosening and removal of phlegm from the respiratory tract

Flatulence -- State of having excessive stomach or intestinal gas

Hypothermia -- Condition in which an organism's temperature drops below that required for normal metabolism and bodily functions

Nervine -- Strengthens functional activity of nervous system – may be stimulants or sedatives

Rubefacient -- Stimulates blood flow to the skin, causing local reddening

Sedative -- Agent that exerts a soothing or tranquilizing effect

Stimulant -- Agent that increases internal heat, dispels internal chill and strengthens metabolism and circulation

Thermogenic -- Agent that produces heat in the body

Tonic -- Agent that exerts a gentle strengthening effect on the body

REFERENCES

LINK 1:
https://www.betterhealth.vic.gov.au/health/healthyliving/anger-how-it-affects-people
http://www.webmd.com/mental-health/tc/seasonal-affective-disorder-sad-topic-overview

http://www.beliefnet.com/wellness/articles/the-toxic-effect-of-guilt.aspx

Elena Patrick (2014), "How's Your Emotional Health, How to Enhance Your Mental Wellness and Emotional Health Now", Chapter 2 "What Is Emotional Health". Kindle Edition

Virtue, Doreen, PhD (2002), "Losing Your Pounds of Pain: Breaking the Link Between Abuse, Stress, and Overeating", Revised Edition pp. 58-70

Hay, Louise, "You Can Heal Your Life", p. 151

https://www.verywell.com/grief-and-mourning-process-1132545?utm_term=physical+symptoms+of+grief&utm_content=p1-main-7-

LINK 2:
http://faculty.washington.edu/chudler/auto.html

https://en.wikipedia.org/wiki/Parasympathetic_nervous_system

https://en.wikipedia.org/wiki/Sympathetic_nervous_system

http://www.innerbody.com/image/musfov.html
http://www.livestrong.com/article/88742-three-types-muscles-human-body/

Yoshida, Cynthia M., MD (2004), "No More Digestive Problems", pp. 254-257

Thibodeau, Gary A., PhD and Patton, Kevin T., PhD (2000); "Structure and Function of the Human Body", Eleventh Edition, pp. 59-70, Chapter 16, p. 403 and p. 411

LINK 3:
"Your Body Type: Find Out Why It Matters", Kindle version

http://www.diabetes.co.uk/body/visceral-fat.html

http://www.muscleandstrength.com/articles/body-types-ectomorph-mesomorph-endomorph.html

LINK 4:
"The Complete Master Cleanse, A Step by Step Guide to the Lemonade Diet" by Tom Woloshyn
http://www.drugwarfacts.org/cms/Causes_of_Death

Hobbs, Christopher, L.Ac (2002), "Natural Therapy for Your Liver" Revised and Updated; Herbs and Other Natural Remedies for a Healthy Liver"

Haas, Elson M., M.D., (1992), "Staying Healthy with Nutrition". Pp. 408-409, 522-523, 534-536

Liver Enriching Foods: http://www.hepatitis.org.uk/s-crina/liver-f3-main3.htm

http://www.hepatitis.org.uk/s-crina/liver-f3-main3.htm

LINK 5:
http://www.livestrong.com/article/153409-what-are-the-most-toxic-vitamins/

http://www.livestrong.com/article/448407-how-are-fat-soluble-vitamins-absorbed/

https://medlineplus.gov/ency/article/002410.htm

https://www.verywell.com/the-benefits-of-biotin-88316?utm_term=biotin+side+effects+in+women&utm_content=p1-main-1-

Vitamins and Minerals Made Easy: Drastically Improve Your Life With a Few Simple Steps by Gordon Green (ebook)

http://www.ehow.com/info_8795108_difference-micro-minerals-macro-minerals.html

BACK TO EDEN by Jethro Kloss – pp. 457-541

LINK 6:
http://internalharmony.com/articles/14/Lymphatic-System-What-is-it.html
"Immune Boost – Total Aegis: Best Ways to Fortify Your Body's Defenses" by Lucas Ester

LINK 7:
http://www.chatelaine.com/health/diet/tired-overweight-you-might-be-too-acidic/

Young, Robert O. PhD; Young, Shelley Redford (2005), "The pH Miracle of Weight Loss"

LINK 8:
"Complete Food Combining, All You Need to Know About the Hay Diet" by Peter Thomson (Kindle Edition)

LINK 9:
The Little Herb Encyclopedia, The Handbook of Nature's Remedies for a Healthier Life, Third Edition, Jack Ritchason, ND, Copyright 1995, Published by Woodland Health Books: pp. 5-153; pp. 206-214; pp. 235-263
Prescription for Herbal Healing, pp. 14-149

The Humorous Herbalist, pp. 28-34, pp. 47-51, pp. 58-63, pp. 73-79, pp. 86-91, pp. 128-132

Nutritional Herbology, A Reference Guide to Herbs, Revised and Expanded Edition, Mark Pedersen, Copyright 1998, Published by Wendell W. Whitman Company

PDR for Herbal Medicines, First Edition, Medical Economics Company, New York

The New Age Herbalist, Consulting Editor Richard Mabey, et al, Published by Simon & Schuster Inc., Copyright 1988 by Gaia Books Ltd., London

http://www.ncbi.nlm.nih.gov/pubmed/11035521?dopt=Abstract

LINK 10:
Batmanghelidj, F., M.D. (1992). "Your Body's Many Cries for Water", Second Edition, pp.13, 48-49

LINK 11:
"The 10 Day Skin Brushing Detox" by Mia Campbell, Kindle Edition

LINK 12:
"Rebounding on A Mini-Trampoline" by Christopher David Allen (Kindle Edition)

LINK 13:
www.merriam-webster.com

"Zapped" by Anne Louise Gittleman

LINK 14:
"Secrets of Bach Flower Remedies by Dr. Ketki S. Itraj" ebook on Kindle

"Bach Flower Remedies" by Shalini Kagal (Kindle Edition 2013)

LINK 15:
PDR (People's Desk Reference) for Essential Oils – Compiled by Essential Science Publishing

LINK 16:
Body Reflexology, Healing At Your Fingertips by Mildred Carter and Tammy Weber

Better Health with Reflexology by Dwight Byers

Kunz, Barbara; Kunz, Kevin. Medical Applications of Reflexology, RRP Press. Kindle Edition.